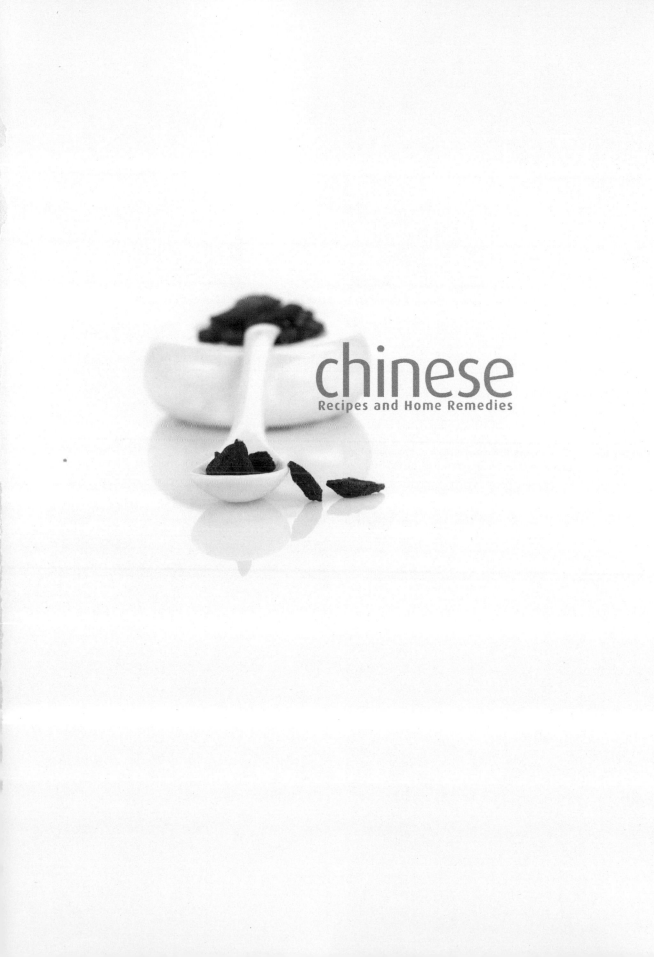

chinese
Recipes and Home Remedies

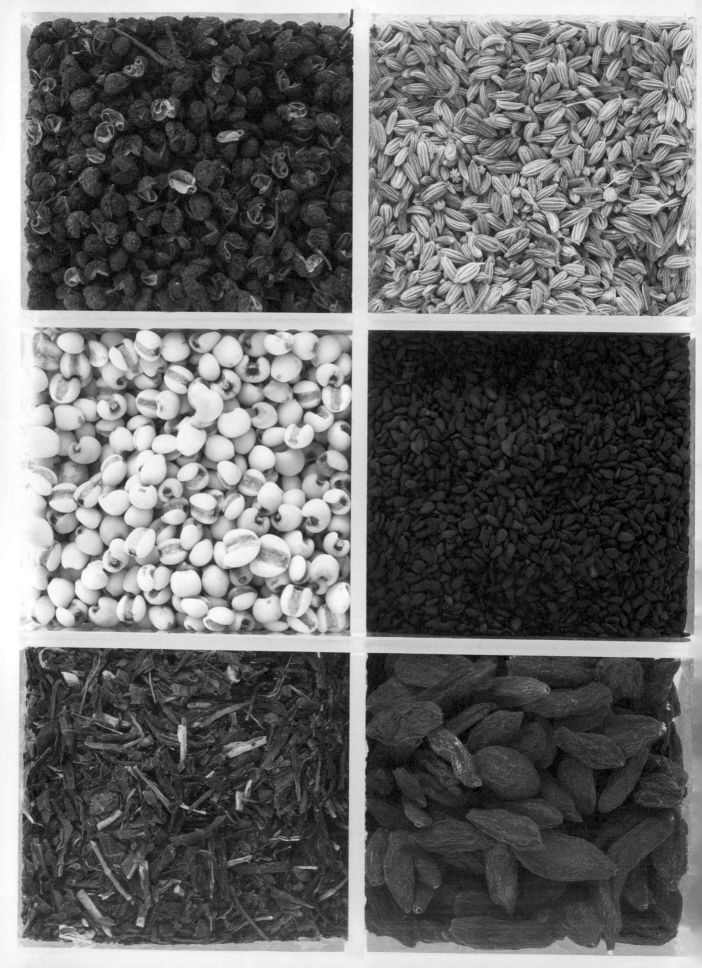

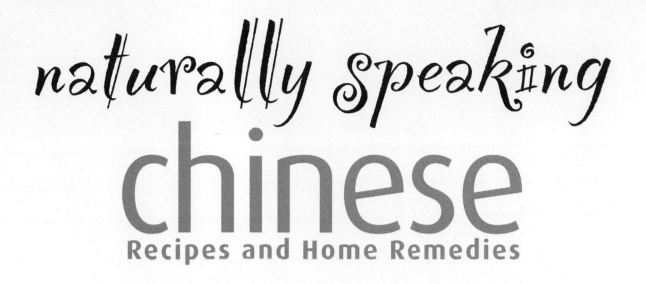

naturally speaking
chinese
Recipes and Home Remedies

Terry Tan

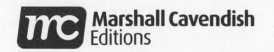

Marshall Cavendish
Editions

The publisher wishes to thank Dragon Brand Bird's Nest for the use of their bird's nest, ginseng and cordyceps for the photography of this book.

Editor : Selina Lim Siew Lin
Designer : Bernard Go Kwang Meng
Photographer : Joshua Tan, Elements by the Box
Food Preparation : Christopher Tan
Model : Ang Chiew Ting

© 2007 Marshall Cavendish International (Asia) Private Limited

Published by Marshall Cavendish Editions
An imprint of Marshall Cavendish International
1 New Industrial Road, Singapore 536196

This publication represents the opinions and views of the author based on his personal experience, knowledge and research. The information in this book is not intended for use in place of proper medical advice. Persons with medical conditions should consult qualified physicians before starting any form of treatment. The author and publisher have used their best efforts in preparing this book and disclaim liability rising directly or indirectly from the use and application of this book.

Other Marshall Cavendish Offices:
Marshall Cavendish Ltd. 119 Wardour Street, London W1F 0UW, UK • Marshall Cavendish Corporation. 99 White Plains Road, Tarrytown NY 10591-9001, USA • Marshall Cavendish International (Thailand) Co Ltd. 253 Asoke, 12th Flr, Sukhumvit 21 Road, Klongtoey Nua, Wattana, Bangkok 10110, Thailand • Marshall Cavendish (Malaysia) Sdn Bhd, Times Subang, Lot 46, Subang Hi-Tech Industrial Park, Batu Tiga, 40000 Shah Alam, Selangor Darul Ehsan, Malaysia

Marshall Cavendish is a trademark of Times Publishing Limited.

National Library Board Singapore Cataloguing in Publication Data

Tan, Terry.
Chinese recipes and home remedies / Terry Tan. – Singapore : Marshall Cavendish Editions, c2007.
p. cm. – (Naturally speaking)
ISBN-13 : 978-981-232-717-8
ISBN-10 : 981-232-717-7

1. Medicine, Chinese. 2. Cookery, Chinese. 3. Cookery (Herbs)
4. Functional foods. I. Title. II. Series: Naturally speaking

TX724.5.C5
641.5951 -- dc22   SLS2007009475

Printed in China by Everbest Printing Co Ltd

Acknowledgements

The author offers grateful thanks to:

Christopher Tan for his cooking and brilliant styling concepts;

Dr. Geng Yu Ling (TCM practitioner) for her professional advice and recipe ideas;

Joshua Tan for his inspiring photography.

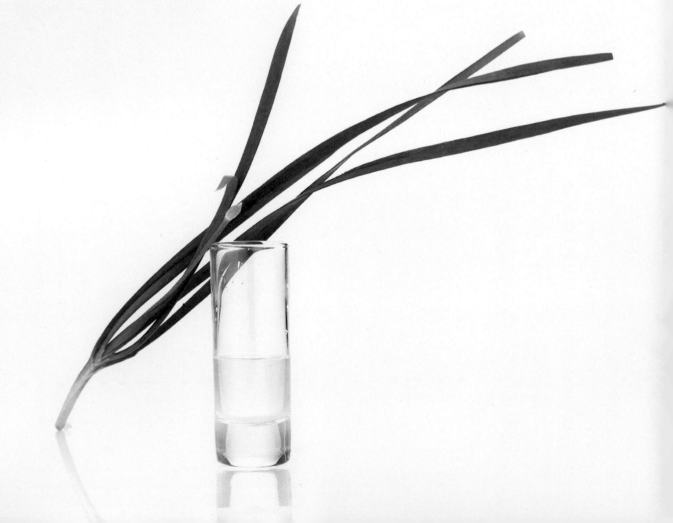

Introduction

When I was approached to do this book, my initial reaction was, how would I justify another book of herbs and spices that is far removed from my previous book, *Cooking with Chinese Herbs*? Huddling with my first editor Selina Kuo, we thrashed out the nuts and bolts for this new book, and concluded that both books would be complementary rather than repetitive. The point is that herbs and spices, whether fresh or dried, and of vegetable origin, have been humanity's culinary mainstays since time immemorial.

It is irrefutable that to maintain good health, we must eat foods that contain the necessary nutritive and bactericidal properties. More so today, when we know that herbs and spices not only flavour and improve the taste of our food, but supply us with nutritional and prophylactic elements.

Accounts of the use of herbs — a term that embraces the spectrum of plants, rhizomes, fruits, vegetables, seeds, barks etc — can be traced back to 2500 b.c. in China, as well as the Mediterranean countries, India and tropical Asia. The ancient texts that form the basis of Traditional Chinese Medicine (TCM) are still studied and followed by practitioners the world over. TCM is an ancient and time-honoured discipline that is universal and understands the efficacy of a multitude of herbs, barks, roots, nuts and seeds.

It was Hippocrates, the Father of Greek medicine who said, 'Let food be your medicine and medicine be your food.'

The sage may have been the father of medicine but, long before his existence, in the 2nd century of medieval Europe, there was a physician named Galen who had classified herbs by their essential qualities of 'hot' or 'cold', 'dry' or 'damp'. This was not far removed from the principles of Chinese herbalism. By the 7th century, Arab physicians had elaborated these Galenical findings and established what was called Unani medicine, still practised in the Muslim world and India.

In any dissertation on herbalism, one cannot avoid reference to the other Asian branch of medicine, Ayurveda. The name comes from two ancient Indian words, 'ayur' meaning life, and 'veda', which means knowledge. Like TCM, Ayurveda sees illness as imbalance, and herbs are prescribed to restore the necessary equilibrium. And the discipline goes back as far as TCM does, to 2500 b.c. Successive dynasties and invaders added to the store of knowledge, including the Persians in 500 b.c. and the Moghuls in the 14th century. In more recent times, Tibetan medicine, that has much in common with Ayurveda, has also exerted some influences.

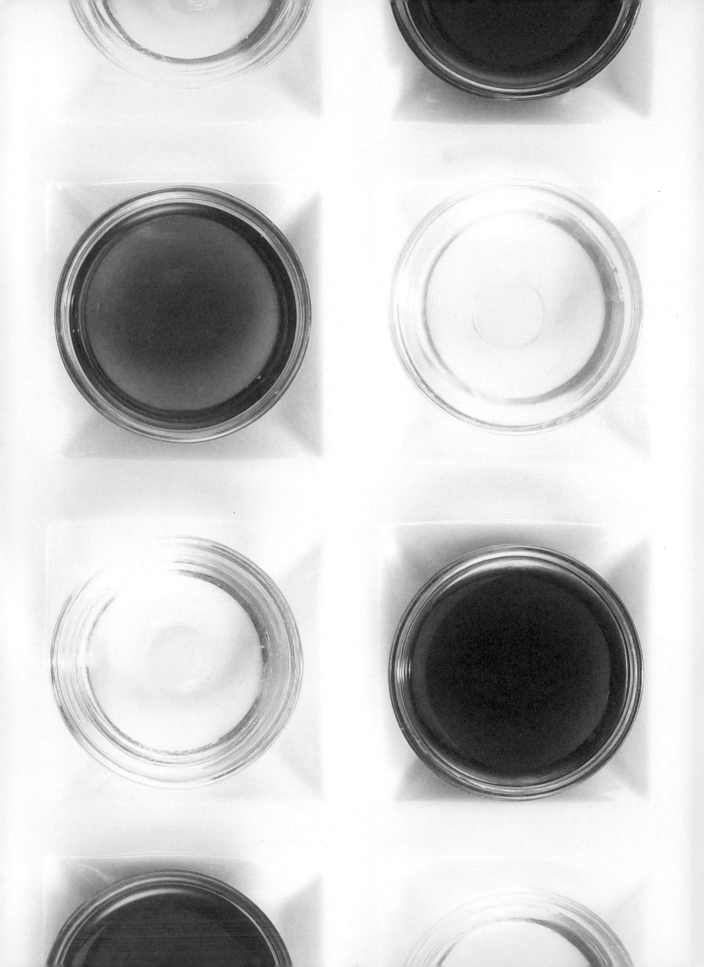

The Principles of Traditional Chinese Medicine (TCM)

In antiquity, people who considered themselves medical thinkers, were theoreticians rather than practitioners; they rarely saw patients. Much of the healing was left to local elderly women with no academic training, but who were custodians of handed-down remedies. During the Han dynasty 2000 years ago, the idea mooted in regard to human ills was that there had to be correct balance between all the parts of a human body. The concept of Qi or Energy was initiated, to be followed by acupuncture. Herbal remedies were used therapeutically within this belief.

The idea of correct balance between all parts of the human body, along with the concept of Qi, acupuncture and herbal healing are based on the 'theory of five elements', that explains all the interactions between humanity and its environment. They are namely Wood, Fire, Earth, Metal and Water, all seen to be related, as in wood fueling fire, the earth being resolved by fire and yielding metal that produces water (condensation on a cold surface) and water feeding vegetation to produce wood.

It is important to first understand the semantics of Chinese culture and thought processes, in order to place TCM in the right context. Existence is dependent on three fundamentals in the culture: Jing refers to the substance of all living organisms. Then there is Shen, which embodies spirit, thought and consciousness. Between Jing and Shen is Qi or Chi. While some westerners and even medical practitioners airily dismiss Qi as a somewhat unreal entity, it is the very embodiment of health and well-being. This is probably because much of it is beyond scientific validation and clinical definition. Many Chinese herbs today have been validated by medical authorities worldwide. Fundamentally, Qi is the body's vital energy that flows in a network of channels or meridians that can be stimulated with acupuncture.

In essence, there are three types of Jing:

GENETIC characteristics that predetermine a person's constitution. This is not that far removed from the western concept of genetically predetermined characteristics, like inherited ailments of diabetes, haemophilia and hypertension.

SUSTENANCE the intake of food and the state of the body's digestive system.

AIR that we breathe and closely related to the functions of the lungs.

Therefore, the diagnosis of the human condition is dependent upon the state of a patient's Qi in all its manifestations. Hence, a Chinese herbalist will look at a patient's tongue firstly to determine many things: that the liver is not functioning well, or that he or she has too much Yang 'heat' etc. The objective is to prescribe the correct herbal mix, either as a medicinal brew, or to be ingested with food to forge a better balance of Qi.

There are also many other complementary aspects to be considered in treatment. Is the patient suffering from 'excess heat' that causes fever and extreme thirst in the patient, or 'dampness', which leads to the production of excess phelgm in his or her system? Is there deficiency or excess of one or the other characteristic? Conditions like stagnation, blood circulation and resistance within and without the body, are all taken into studied account before any diagnosis is made. In short, the herbalist will build up a picture of where the imbalances are, before prescribing the necessary counteraction. It is more to do with how each herbal mix will affect the imbalances than the chemical constituents it contains.

In essence, Chinese herbalism relies little on technology, but on the classification of different herbs according to how they influence characteristics. The yardstick is really the different 'tastes' of herbal remedies of which there are five that relate to human responses.

The Five Tastes

PUNGENCY Related to the lungs, this dispels stagnation and promotes circulation and movement. It is applied when there is deficiency in body heat, and is associated with a hot, acrid taste, as in pepper and chillies.

SWEET Related to the stomach and classified as a warming element, it is nutritionally tonifying and less extreme than pungency.

SALTY Associated with the kidneys, water and cooling influences, to help soften or moisten tissues that suffer from excessive dryness, for example, gargling with salted warm water for sore throats.

BITTER Associated with the heart, 'coolness' and 'dryness', this is extreme action that stimulates the taste buds and helps to improve sluggish digestion, and ward off fevers.

SOUR Classified as the most neutral of the 'five tastes' and not associated with either 'hot' or 'cooling' actions, this flavour is related to the liver and astringent ingredients like tea and citrus fruits.

Yin and Yang

This theory of opposites complements the fundamental 'five elements' and denotes that everything in the cosmos contains, and is balanced by, its polar opposite. The Yin Yang theory has long since informed Chinese thought and beliefs, although some atheist views still persist and regard it as mystical hokum. In traditional Chinese culture, indeed in life itself, everything boils down to the opposite forces of Yin and Yang. The former, in broad strokes, represents the earth, moon, female gender and darkness, as well as the negative principles of coldness, passivity and softness. The latter, at the other end of the spectrum, represents the sun, heaven, male gender and light, as well as properties such as heat, activity and hardness.

Any imbalance is therefore the pointer to a patient's state of health and this is where the two complementary aspects come into play. Unlike the western notion of health, a balanced diet, according Chinese herbalists, does not rest on the correct amounts of proteins, vitamins, fats and sugars. It is the balance of the body's Qi elements that ensures this status quo. Broadly speaking, Yin represents the material substance of a person and Yang is related to energy or dynamic function.

Thus, a person harbouring elements of a state of 'coldness' can counter the condition by eating 'hot' foods and, likewise, elements of 'heat' can be countered by drinking 'cooling' brews, or by taking medicinal brews made from 'cold' herbs. Therefore, the ultimate and deceptively simple objective is to strike a perfect balance between the opposing forces by aiding their mutual interaction and maintain good health.

Most foods are also classified either Yin or Yang according to the 'five elements', and in relation to the 'five tastes'. There is also the important relation of food to particular organs and acupuncture meridians, just as for herbs. The foods that are deemed 'cool', bitter and salty are more Yin, while 'hot', sweet and pungent foods are Yang. Most fruits are classified Yin

The state of Yin can also be adversely affected by hot, humid conditions and therefore, more Yin foods like melons and cucumber can give Yin energies a push. Personalities are also classified in similar fashion. Someone who can withstand cold, and is prone to heaty problems like mouth ulcers and boils, is generally Yang and should eat more cold, bitter foods like celery and bitter gourd, and avoid chillies and hot curries.

Glossary

Throughout this book, you will come across various terms that describe the healing properties of the herbs, spices and other ingredients. The following is a useful guide for your easy reference.

ANODYNE any herb or spice that acts as a natural painkiller.

ANTISPASMODIC muscular cramps, spasms and contractions need the help of herbs that have antispasmodic action to help relax muscles.

AROMATIC applied mostly to scented herbs and spices that are generally good for improving digestion.

ASTRINGENT associated mainly with substances that contain tannic acids. They contract, firm and strengthen skin and other tissue. Also used in the treatment of inflammation.

CATHARTIC refers to substances that induce purging, especially from the digestive system.

DEMULCENT substances that provide a soothing effect on the digestive tract and exterior dermis. Mucilages contain this action as they form a 'skin' on the infected area, allowing it to heal while being protected.

EXPECTORANT closely associated with any herbal remedy that aids coughs. It helps to loosen thick phlegm so that the phlegm can be coughed up easily.

LAXATIVE works by increasing activity in the bowel, or by softening and lubricating hard stools.

NERVINE works on the nervous system and covers a fairly wide range of remedies. While some are stimulating, others are relaxing and the main action is in the strengthening of nerves.

TONIC in general, it applies to those herbs that nourish, stimulate or strengthen the different functions of the body.

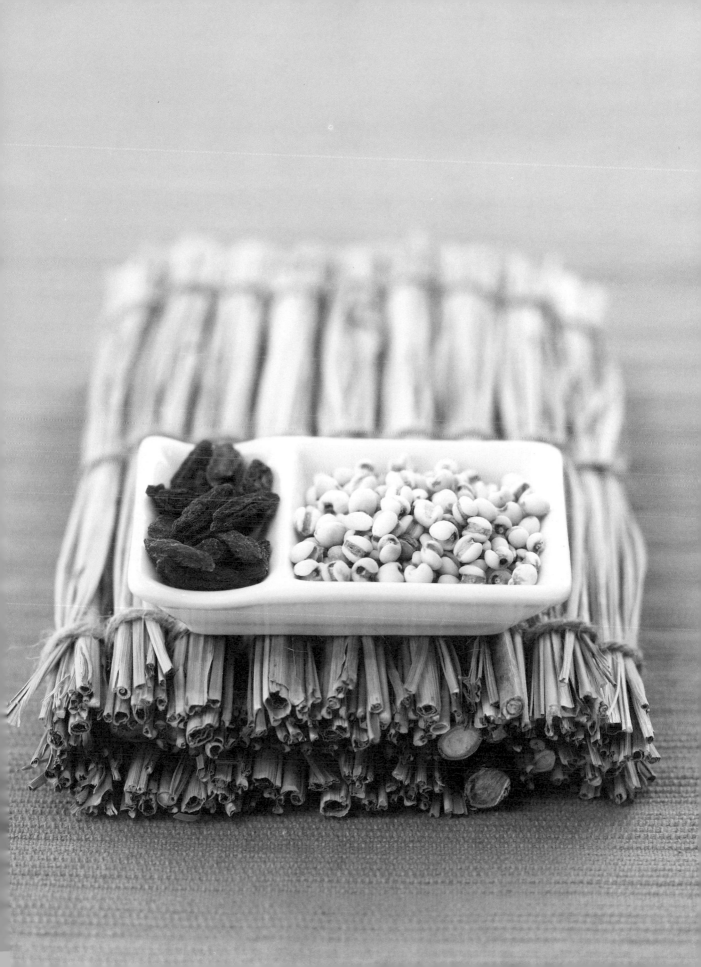

Aloe Vera

This must be the miracle plant of mankind and one that is increasingly ubiquitous and manifest in an astonishing range of products from drinks to shampoos, all using its gel — the translucent, gummy remains of aloe vera leaves after their hard, green outer layers are removed.

Common Aloe vera
Mandarin Lu hui
Cantonese Lohr wai
Botanical Aloe barbadensies

I have had, for the past 20 years, several aloe vera plants in my garden that I have used extensively. As aloe vera juice is cathartic, it is inadvisable to consume it while using medication. Aloe vera gel, however, is one of nature's most wonderful healing substances. I eat its sap au naturel, apply it on cuts and sores and generally treat it as an extremely good intestinal cleanser and mild laxative. Chinese herbalists use it to aid intestinal and stomach functions, kill parasites and neutralise toxins. Aloe vera is also excellent for the treatment of joint aches and pains, headaches and fever and ringworm infestations. You can cultivate the plant easily as long as it is kept indoors when there is frost. Otherwise, it is very self-sufficient, requiring a little water on very hot days and will reward you with many new shoots when happy. It is also a very pretty indoor plant as a potted succulent.

Aloe Vera and Kalamansi Quencher

Preparation time: 10 minutes
Serves 4

The cooling drink is one of my summer favourites.

Kalamansi limes 6	Halve limes and squeeze for juice. Add juice to water and stir to mix, then set aside.
Water 800 ml (26 fl oz / 3¼ cups)	
Sugar 2 Tbsp	Dissolve sugar thoroughly in a little water. Heat in a microwave oven, or briefly over stove-top, if required.
Fresh aloe vera gel 2 Tbsp, cubed	
Ice cubes 8 cubes, crushed	Add dissolved sugar and aloe vera gel to lime juice solution, stir through and pour over crushed ice.
Lime slices for garnish (optional)	
	Garnish each drink, if desired, with lime slices.

FROM LEFT TO RIGHT: *Aloe Vera and Kalamansi Quencher (page 15), Aloe Agar Agar (page 16)*

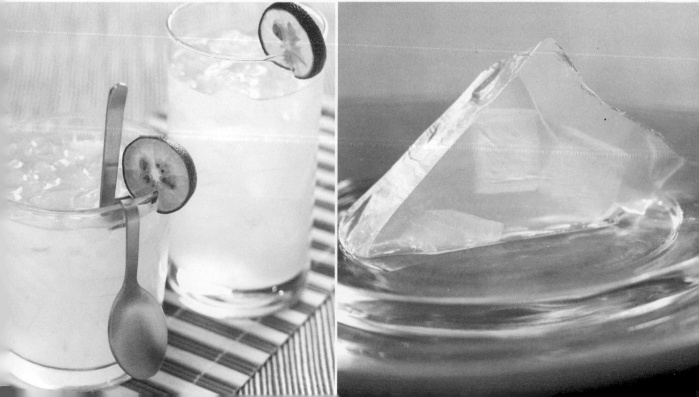

Aloe Agar-agar

I chanced upon this hybrid while testing Japanese agar-agar one day and thought, why not an aloe infusion? It works well as the two products have perfect synergy. I used the gel straight from the plant, but it is commercially available too.

Preparation time: 10 minutes
Cooking time: 20 minutes
Serves 4

Agar-agar powder 15 g (^{1}/$_2$ oz)

Konnyaku powder 15 g (^{1}/$_2$ oz)

Caster (superfine) sugar 140 g (5 oz)

Water 800 ml (25^1/$_3$ fl oz / 3^1/$_4$ cups)

Screwpine (*pandan*) leaf 1, knotted

Fresh aloe vera gel 250 g (9 oz), cut into small dice

Combine agar-agar and konnyaku powders and sugar in a pot. Gradually whisk in water.

When all the water has been added, add screwpine leaf and bring mixture to the boil over medium heat, stirring constantly. Reduce heat and simmer gently for 5 minutes, whisking constantly to make sure all the powder dissolves.

Remove and discard screwpine leaf. Stir in aloe vera dice, then immediately ladle mixture into jelly moulds. Leave to cool completely, then refrigerate until chilled and set.

When set, cut into desired shapes and serve as a dessert.

Note: Konnyaku and agar-agar are gelling agents that lend different properties to this jelly; konnyaku adds translucency while agar-agar adds firmness and stability. The result pleasantly mimics the texture of aloe vera.

Treatments

If you cultivate aloe vera as a house plant, cut off a thick, mature leaf every so often and scrape off the gel with a spoon. Eat it as it is and let the constituents do the work for a whole range of abdominal problems. Fresh aloe vera gel can also be applied directly on sunburn, burns, cuts and wounds to accelerate the healing process.

Aromatherapy

Aloe vera essential oil is a penetrating moisturiser that is naturally hypoallergenic and one of the few natural ingredients that has more or less the same pH as human skin. It is an excellent massage oil when mixed with a carrier or base oil, such as almond or apricot oil. This blend is astringent and anti-fungal with rejuvenating properties. The oil is known to relieve arthritis and stimulate the immune system.

Beauty

Make your own **aloe facial mask** for a real smooth complexion. Simply blend 1 Tbsp aloe vera gel with 2 Tbsp thick natural yoghurt and use as a face pack. Leave for 15 minutes before rinsing off.

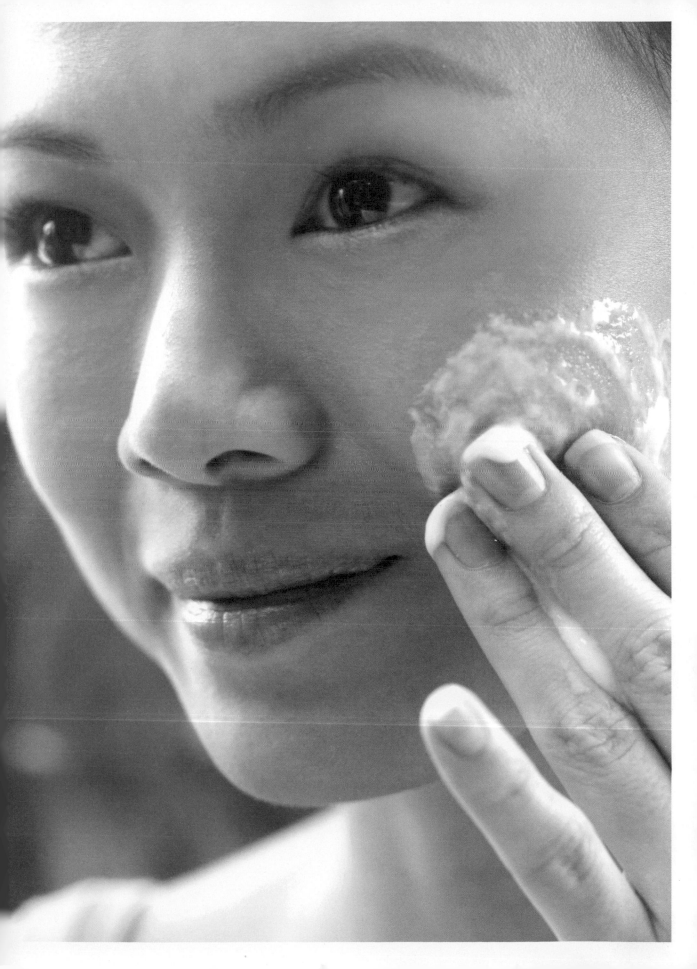

Apricot Kernel

Common Apricot kernel
Mandarin Xing ren
Cantonese Hung ngan
Botanical Prunus armeniaca semen

Hung ngan, the kernel of a Mongolian apricot, is also found in Manchuria and the northern provinces of Hebei, Beijing and Shandong in north China. The creamy-white kernels are better known as Chinese almonds even though they are extracted from the hard stones of apricots.

In Korea, it is used as an expectorant and a remedy for dry throat, laryngitis and lung diseases. In China and Japan, it is regarded as a sedative for respiratory problems, a tonic and remedy for severe colds, asthma, rheumatism, swollen feet and constipation, while in Vietnam, a special preparation of the smashed fruit is chewed but not swallowed, to protect the bronchial tubes from cold during winter. Nevertheless, their flavour is remarkably similar to that of true, brown-skinned almonds. Chinese herbal shops always stock two varieties of apricot kernels — sweet and bitter. The former are smaller and rounder, and are also known as 'southern almonds' to the Chinese; *nan xing* in Mandarin and *nam hung* in Cantonese. The latter are larger and flatter, and called 'northern almonds' by the Chinese, or *bei xing* in Mandarin and *puk hung* in Cantonese. The two types are typically used in equal proportions in Chinese herbal recipes.

Apricot Kernels with White Fungus and Gingko Nuts

This blend makes for a soothing brew that helps to clear the lungs and dispel phlegm. Drink it twice a week until the ailment is cured.

Preparation time: 10 minutes
Cooking time: 45 minutes
Serves 4

White fungus 55 g (2 oz)
Sweet apricot kernels 20 g (²/₃ oz)
Bitter apricot kernels 20 g (²/₃ oz)
Water 1 litre (32 fl oz / 4 cups)
Precooked gingko nuts 40 g (1¹/₃ oz)
Rock sugar 140 g (5 oz)

Soak white fungus in plenty of water and cut into smaller pieces. Rinse, drain well and set aside.

Place apricot kernels in a colander and rinse well, then drain and set aside.

Combine water, apricot kernels, white fungus and gingko nuts in a pot. Bring to the boil and simmer over low heat for 45 minutes, adding water as necessary.

Add rock sugar and simmer until completely dissolved. Remove from heat. Serve hot or chilled, as desired.

Treatments

Creams and lotions processed from apricot kernels make effective moisturisers, and have a reputation for improving skin tone.

Aromatherapy

Apricot oil is a carrier or base oil, rich with oleic and linoleic acids that are easily absorbed into the skin. It does not have a strong aroma and is usually combined with small amounts of essential oils to become a more usable product, such as a massage oil. Without the carrier oil, essential oils will evaporate rapidly. Apricot oil makes an excellent massage oil as it is not too greasy and leaves the skin feeling silky smooth.

Apricot Kernels with White Fungus and Gingko Nuts (page 19)

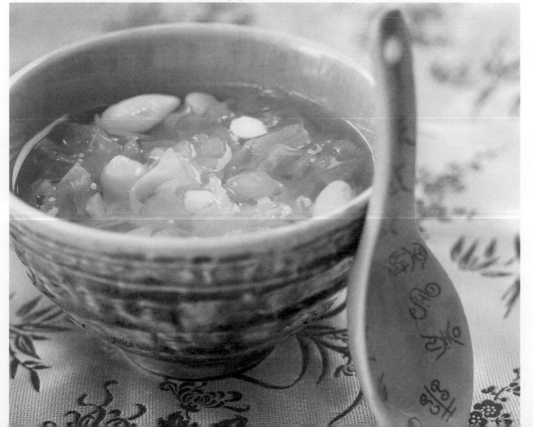

Astragalus Root

Found in Korea and the provinces of Shanxi and Gansu in China, astragalus roots have brown skins and are pale yellow inside. Usually sold dried and ready-sliced into thin slivers, the root is found to be a potent stimulant of the immune system. In TCM, it is believed to increase white blood cells and is commonly used for the treatment of poor blood circulation and fatigue. The warming action of the herb also influences lung and spleen functions, benefits Qi circulation and reduces water retention. It is effective in the treatment of excessive perspiration, severe blood loss, oedema and chronic sores.

Common Astragalus root
Mandarin Huang qi
Cantonese Puk kei
Botanical Astragalus membranaceus

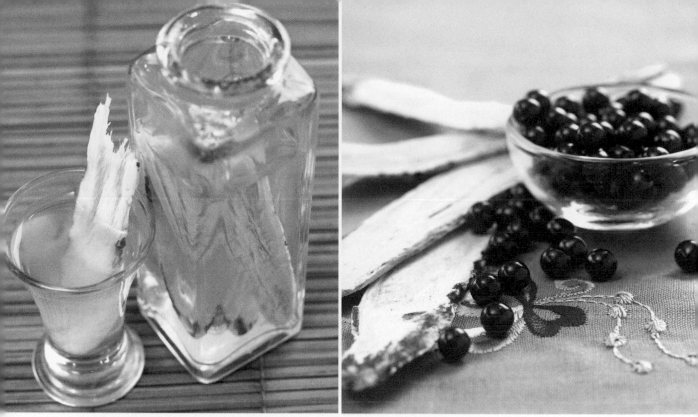

FROM LEFT TO RIGHT: Astragalus Wine (page 21), Treatment: Astragalus Pills for Balancing Qi (page 22)

Astragalus and Codonopsis Tea

Herbal medicine researchers have recorded that codonopsis root can increase the number of red corpuscles and reduce the number of leucocytes in the blood. The root has, on occasion, been mistakenly identified as the mid-section of ginseng. Astragalus and codonopsis, when combined, help to soothe throat problems and revitalise sagging energy.

Preparation time: 10 minutes
Cooking time: 35 minutes
Serves 4

Astragalus root 15 g (¹/₂ oz), rinsed and drained

Codonopsis root 15 g (¹/₂ oz), rinsed and drained

Rock sugar 50 g (2 oz)

Water 800 ml (26 fl oz / 3¹/₄ cups)

Combine all ingredients in a pot. Bring to the boil and simmer over medium heat for about 35 minutes.

Remove from heat and serve as desired.

Note: You may add a handful of pitted Chinese red dates for a slightly sweeter flavour.

Astragalus Wine (Huang Qi Jiu)

My Chinese herbalist-advisor, Dr Geng Yu-ling, tells me this is a marvellous tipple for when you feel your Qi is less than perfect, or when you are suffering from weak limbs and breathlessness. It is ever so simple to make and really nice to drink, in moderation, of course.

Preparation time: 10 minutes

Astragalus root 110 g (4 oz) rinsed and drained, pat dry with paper towels thoroughly

Chinese rice wine or sake 500 ml (16 fl oz / 2 cups)

Place astragalus root in a clean glass bottle with wine or sake, and steep for a month. Shake gently every week.

Strain wine into a clean jar and discard herb. Cork and serve at room temperature or slightly warmed, if using sake.

Chicken with Astragalus Root and Chinese Wolfberries

Chinese wolfberries have a delicately sweet flavour that is almost imperceptible. As a rough guide, use a handful or about 2 Tbsp for an amount of soup for 4 persons.

Preparation time: 15 minutes
Cooking time: 1 hour
Serves 4

Chicken 900 g (2 lb),
   or 600 g (1 lb 5 oz) lean pork

Astragalus root 15 g ($^1/_2$ oz),
   rinsed and drained

Chinese wolfberries 2 Tbsp,
   rinsed and drained

Water 1.5 litres (48 fl oz / 6 cups)

Salt 2 tsp

Black pepper to taste

Fresh coriander leaves (cilantro)
   for garnish

Clean chicken and leave whole. If preferred, cut into large joints and remove excess fatty skin. If using pork, cut cleaned meat into bite-sized chunks.

Combine all ingredients in a pot and simmer for about 1 hour, or until meat is tender.

Serve hot. For an added fillip, sprinkle your soup with pepper to taste, and garnish with coriander leaves.

Note: You will find that chicken meat is rendered rather bland after prolonged simmering, but there is no reason not to eat it, dipped in soy or chilli sauce for good measure.

Treatments

According to TCM, the skin is a sensitive organ that can suffer imbalances due to stress or poor diet. When the body tries to expel the impurities resulting from these imbalances through the skin, pimples and acne result. **Astragalus pills for balancing Qi** are great for nourishing the skin by clearing toxins, strengthening the pores and promoting the healing of chronic sores. Astragalus is often used in conjunction with other herbs to produce creams that help to remedy skin infections.

Astragalus and Codonopsis Tea (page 21)

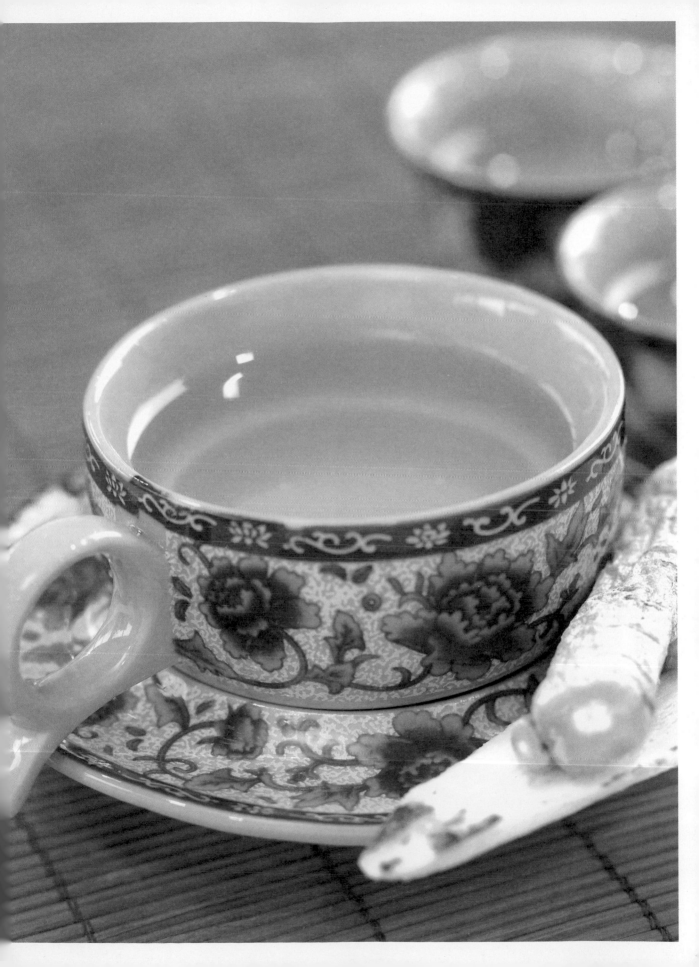

Basil

Common Basil
Mandarin Luo le, Jiu ceng ta
Cantonese Gao chung tahp
Botanical Ocimum basilicum

The basil family is diverse, encompassing different shapes, sizes, colours, aromatic nuances and medicinal promise.

The most common varieties found in Asia are Thai sweet basil, holy basil and lemon basil. In Chinese herbalism, sweet basil is most attributed with healthful qualities. Often referred to simply as basil, it possesses anti-oxidant, as well as anti-inflammatory, analgesic and anti-allergic qualities. The herb is also said to help relieve fever, purge wind, cleanse the blood and strengthen the stomach. To help you identify sweet basil, it has the largest and longest of leaves among its plant family and a mild liquorice-like scent. In Thai herbalism, basil is prescribed for coughs and applied on the skin topically to heal irritations.

Stir-Fried Prawns with Basil and Garlic

As a stir-fried dish, this makes absolutely delicious eating, not to mention its efficacious promise.

Preparation time: 20 minutes
Cooking time: 15 minutes
Serves 4

Tiger prawns (shrimps) 450 g (1 lb)

Sweet basil 20 g (²/₃ oz)

Vegetable oil 2 Tbsp

Garlic 4 cloves, peeled and roughly crushed

Fish sauce 1 Tbsp

Ground black pepper 1 tsp

Sugar 1 tsp

Water 120 ml (4 fl oz / ¹/₂ cup)

Cornflour (cornstarch) 1 Tbsp, mixed with 2 Tbsp water

Shell prawns and devein each one by making a slit along its back with a sharp knife. Wash and drain.

Separate basil leaves from stems and discard fibrous stems. Set aside.

Heat oil and fry garlic for 2 minutes or until golden brown.

Add prawns and stir over high heat for 2 minutes or until prawns are pink.

Add fish sauce, black pepper, sugar and water. Stir over high heat for 1 minute. Thicken with cornflour mixture. Dish out and serve hot with rice and other dishes.

Stir-fried Prawns with Basil and Garlic (page 25)

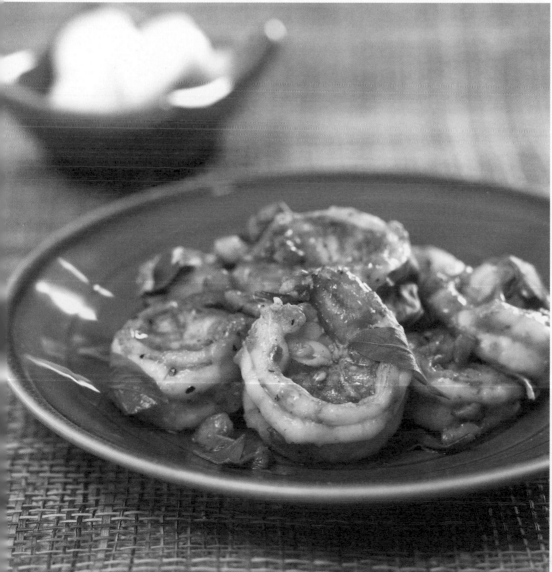

Basil and Egg Drop Soup

This soup is believed to alleviate pre-menstrual pains, gastroenteritis and abdominal swelling.

Preparation time: 10 minutes
Cooking time: 15 minutes
Serves 4

Water 800 ml (26 fl oz / 3¹/₄ cups)

Finely shredded ginger 1 Tbsp

Chinese cooking wine (*shao hsing*) 3 Tbsp, or dry sherry

Light soy sauce 1 Tbsp

Ground black pepper ¹/₂ tsp

Sesame oil 1 Tbsp

Sweet basil 20 g (²/₃ oz)

Eggs 2, lightly beaten

Bring water to the boil in a pot. Add all remaining ingredients, except basil and eggs. Simmer for 5 minutes.

Separate basil leaves from stems and discard fibrous stems. Add leaves to pot and simmer for 3 minutes.

While soup is simmering, pour in beaten egg slowly and stir to make ribbons.

Garnish as desired, and serve hot.

Treatments

Basil cream, available from Chinese herbalists and alternative medicine shops, is a light, greenish-yellow blend that contains linalool — a fragrant liquid typically used in the making of such items as perfumes, soaps and lotions. Also present in such plants as lavender and bergamot, linalool is often used to soothe the skin and render it a certain glow. Not surprising, then, that linalool is a key component in the production of Vitamin E. In TCM, basil is also an important herb in cough medicines and in blends for the treatment of kidney and stomach problems.

Aromatherapy

Basil essential oil is known for its uplifting properties. Add 2–3 drops to an aromatherapy burner, and it will help one to concentrate during long periods of study, or when doing other work that requires mental focus. It has a warm and delicately spiced aroma that is at once, refreshing and rejuvenating. Add a few drops to garden torches at barbecues to dispel midges and other insects too.

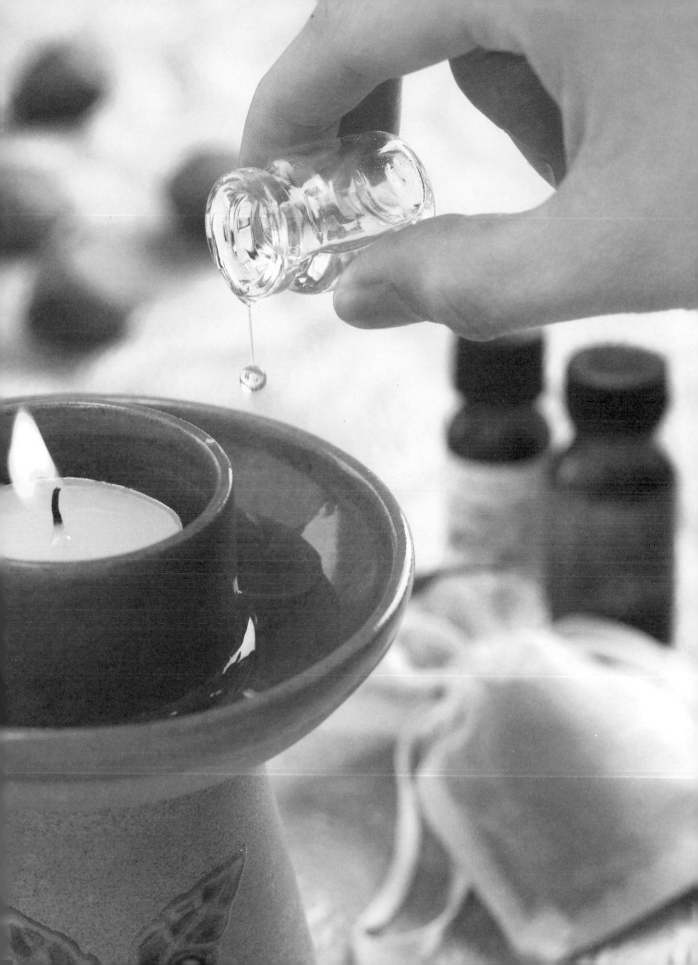

Common Bird's nest
Mandarin Yan wo
Cantonese Yeen wor
Latin Collocal esculenta

Gourmets and other lovers of Chinese cuisine will wax lyrical about bird's nest, but it brings different lumps to different throats. Bird's nests are dried cups of gelatinous, regurgitated saliva with which coastal swallows and swifts line their nests.

The fact that bird's nest can be horrendously expensive probably has everything to do with its inaccessibility. Found mainly in Southeast Asia, the Guangdong province and the plunging fjords of the Fujian province in south China, the swifts' nests are usually found embedded in the deep crevices of dark caves along the coasts.

Whatever the vicissitudes of clambering up and down steep cliffs on bird's-nest-gathering missions, the product of such nerve-wrecking labour is esteemed by millions of Chinese and thousands more of latter-day bird's nest lovers in the western world. Bird's nest is reputed to cleanse the blood of impurities and does wonders for the respiratory system. It also wards off influenza and the common cold. As a delicacy, bird's nest transcends all social barriers. Humble families will buy a little of it to be simmered with not much more than rock sugar and then drunk as a sweet dessert. The more affluent will pay a king's ransom for whole cups of bird's nest and have their cooks prepare sumptuous dishes with poultry and other culinary esoterics.

As with Chinese food products like shark's fin and dried scallops, bird's nest comes in different grades, which, of course, are equated with cost. Since it is not an easy task to differentiate between so-so bird's nest and top-grade cups, one has to rely on the dictum, 'you pay your money and you take your choice'. As a rule of thumb, bird's nest from China is regarded as superior to that from Indonesia and East Malaysia, and the thicker and denser the strands, the better the bird's nest. The highest grade of bird's nest is known as 'blood nest', a pale brown nest speckled with red — believed to be little blood droplets regurgitated by the swifts.

Although bird's nest usually comes nicely cleaned and somewhat bleached in appearance, purists tend to suspect that chemicals may have been added in the process. This accounted for why a lot of younger members of many Chinese families, myself included, used to be marshalled to spend hours picking at twiglets, feathers and other grit from bird's nests which had not been thoroughly cleaned.

Chilled Bird's Nest Drink

For this recipe, the amount of rock sugar can be increased or decreased according to taste. Honey can also be substituted for rock sugar.

Preparation time: 20 minutes
Cooking time: 1–2 hours
Serves 4

Bird's nest 55 g (2 oz)

Rock sugar 140 g (5 oz)

Screwpine (pandan) leaves 2

Water 1 litre (32 fl oz / 4 cups)

Combine all ingredients in a heavy-bottomed or good enamel pot with a snug-fitting lid. Cover and simmer over low heat for 1–2 hours, or until bird's nest is reduced to translucent strips.

Check amount of liquid left in pot every now and then, and top up with water as required.

Remove from heat and leave to cool completely before refrigerating. Serve thoroughly chilled.

Note: To prepare bird's nest that is in its natural state, first use a pair of previously unused or suitably clean tweezers to pick out impurities such as small twigs and tiny feathers, then wash several times. The last change of water should be spotlessly clear.

Chilled Bird's Nest Drink (page 29)

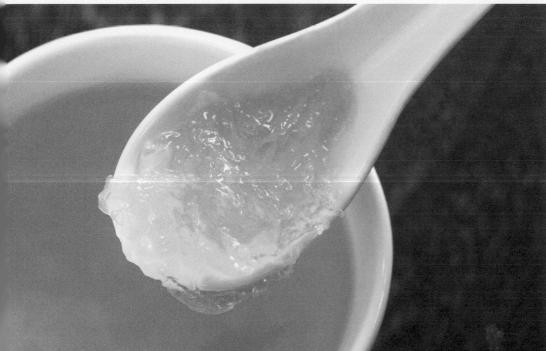

Buddha's Fruit

Buddha's fruit comes from a literal translation of the Mandarin name for the fruit, *luohan* for 'Buddha' and *guo* for 'fruit'.

It is found in Guangxi, Sichuan and Hubei provinces in China. Why it is named after the venerable sage is obscure but reflects the Yin-Yang symbolism of roundness. It is about the size and shape of a kiwi fruit, greenish-brown with a thin shell that crumbles easily. It is good for the treatment of many common ailments including dry coughs, chronic laryngitis and phlegm, as well as other conditions like boils, piles and cramps.

Common Buddha's fruit
Mandarin Luo han guo
Cantonese Lor hawn gor
Botanical Momordica grosvenori

Chicken and Lean Pork Soup with Buddha's Fruit

Buddha's fruit is also known as a longevity herb and is traditionally used for treating mild asthmatic symptoms. The soup becomes a delicious tonic after the meats have been simmered until they are fairly bland, but still edible with a side dip of soy sauce.

Preparation time: 20 minutes
Cooking time: 1 hour
Serves 4–6

Chicken 1, about 900 g (2 lb), cleaned, skinned and trimmed of excess fat

Water 1.5 litres (48 fl oz / 6 cups)

Buddha's fruit 1

Chinese wolfberries 1 Tbsp, rinsed and drained

Lean pork 300 g (11 oz)

Salt 2 tsp

Ground black pepper 1 tsp

Place chicken in a pot with water. Break up Buddha's fruit, rinse and drain.

Add Buddha's fruit to pot with chicken, wolfberries, pork, salt and pepper. Bring to the boil, then simmer over low heat for an hour or so. Strain soup and drink hot.

Note: Although tradition decrees that a whole and very mature bird is used for this recipe, there is no reason why chicken joints cannot be used as they do not bring about a different flavour. If using chicken joints, reduce the cooking time by half.

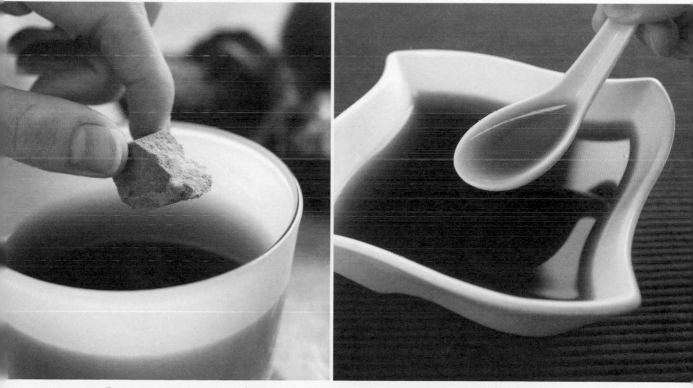

FROM LEFT TO RIGHT: *Treatment:* Lo Han Guo *Sugar Cubes (page 31), Chicken and Lean Pork Soup with Buddha's Fruit (page 31)*

Treatments

Buddha's fruit creams and lotions are used as moisturisers and in the treatment of chloasma, a condition involving skin discolouration in the form of brown spots due to hormonal changes. Typically, a woman is likely to develop such spots during or after pregnancy. Ready-to-use **lo han guo sugar cubes** comprising a mixture of Buddha's fruit and fructose are also available at most Chinese medicinal shops. To use, simply dissolve the sugar cubes in a glass of hot water and drink it for treating coughs, removing excessive phlegm and alleviating heatiness in the body. The natural sugar cubes can also be used to substitute sugar when cooking Chinese sweet soups and drinks.

Cardamom

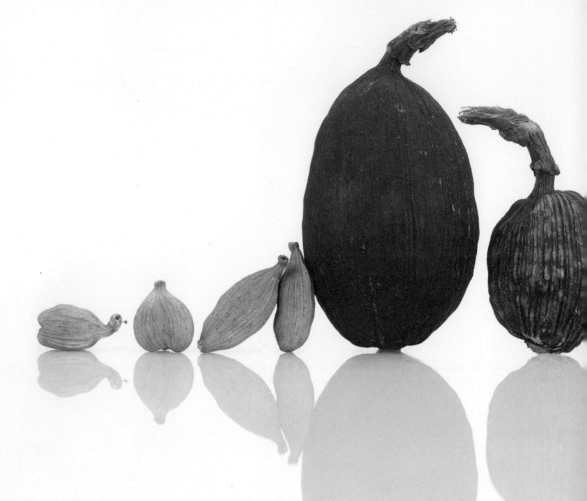

Widely grown in the Middle East, India and Nepal, cardamom comes in two varieties — large black and small green pods. In Ayurvedic medicine, black cardamom are used as stimulants to aid digestion and prevent vomiting. Green cardamoms, on the other hand, are regarded as a cleansing tonic with expectorant and mildly aphrodisiac properties. However, in Chinese herbalism, black cardamom, known as *cao guo,* are more often used for various treatments including warming the kidneys and spleen, as well as treating excessive saliva, diarrhoea and abdominal pains. They have volatile oils and mucilage, accompanied by carminative and diuretic actions.

Although black cardamom are regarded as being the more potent variety of the two in TCM, we give credence to green cardamom which are more universally known. In general, all cardamom help sluggish digestion and prevent flatulence when chewed or brewed with tea.

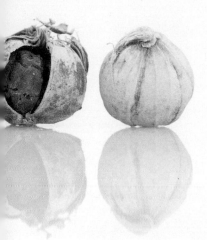

Common Green cardamom, Black cardamom
Mandarin Sha ren, Bai dou kou, Cao guo
Cantonese Bahk dau kau, Chou gwo
Botanical Elettaria cardamomum (Green cardamom),
Amomum subulatum (Black cardamom)

Cardamom, Sweet Basil and Ginger Tea

Preparation time: 5 minutes
Cooking time: 20 minutes
Serves 4

Water 800 ml (26 fl oz / 3 1/4 cup)
Shredded ginger 1 Tbsp
Rock sugar 70 g (2 1/2 oz)
Green cardamom 8 pods
Sweet basil 30 g (1 oz)
Chinese or Indian tea leaves 1 Tbsp

Combine water, ginger, rock sugar and cardamom in a pot. Bring to the boil and simmer for 15 minutes.

Meanwhile, pluck off sweet basil leaves and discard fibrous stems.

After simmering for 15 minutes, add basil leaves and simmer for 3 minutes more.

Add tea leaves, stir through and remove from heat. Leave to steep for 10 minutes. Strain mixture through a fine sieve and transfer to pre-warmed teapot.

Serve hot to improve digestion and relieve flatulence.

Hubei Spicy Chicken

This recipe comes courtesy of my TCM mentor, Dr Geng Yu-ling, who hails from the said northern Chinese province. Like Sichuan and Hunan cooking, Hubei dishes tend to be on the spicy, fiery side, and many soups and stews are characterised by a liberal use of dried spices.

Preparation time: 15 minutes
Cooking time: 45 minutes
Serves 4

Chicken 1, about 1.5 kg (3 lb 4 1/2 oz), cleaned and trimmed of excess fat and skin

Water 1.5 litres (48 fl oz / 6 cups)

Chinese cooking wine (*shao hsing*) 130 ml (4 fl oz / 1/2 cup)

Black cardamom 6 pods

Light soy sauce 1 Tbsp

Dark soy sauce 1 Tbsp

Sichuan peppercorns 1 tsp

Sugar 1 tsp

Cut chicken into 6–8 large joints.

Bring water to the boil in a pot with a snug-fitting lid. Add chicken pieces, wine and cardamom. Cover and simmer for 30 minutes.

Add both soy sauces, peppercorns and sugar. Bring to a rapid boil, uncovered, and continue cooking for another 15 minutes to reduce liquid.

When done, stock should be slightly thick and glossy. Remove from heat and serve immediately with rice.

FROM LEFT TO RIGHT: Hubei Spicy Chicken (page 34), Cardamom, Sweet Basil and Ginger Tea (page 33)

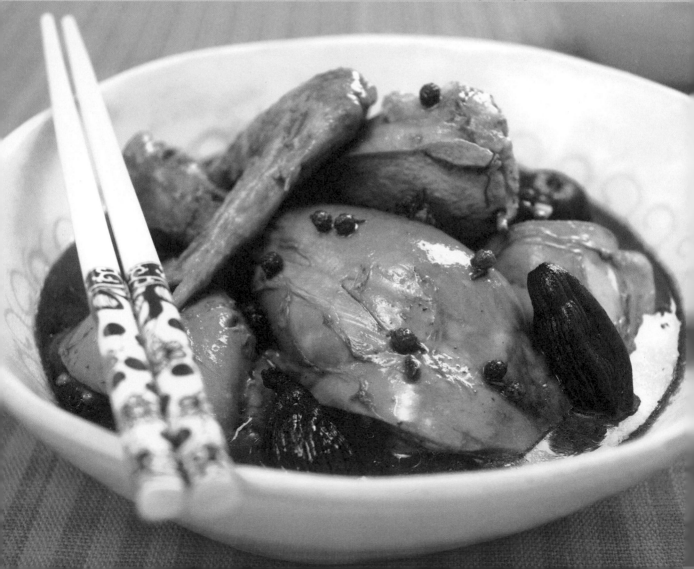

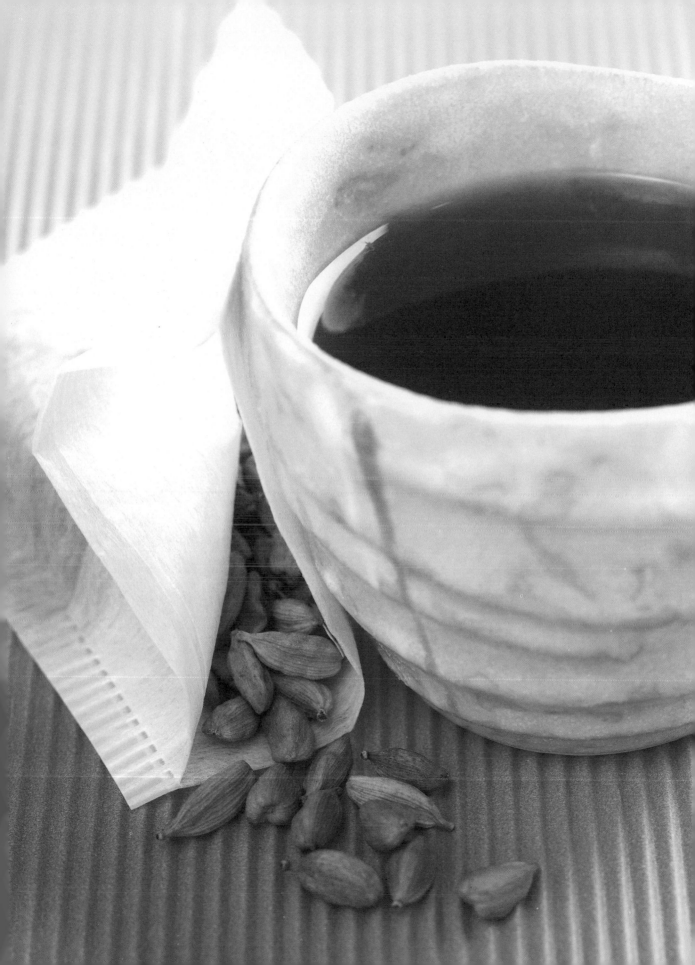

Chinese Angelica

Common Chinese angelica
Mandarin Dang gui
Cantonese Dong quai
Botanical Angelica sinensis

Of the family *umbelliferae*, *dang gui* is recognised as one of the most effective herbal ingredients for a whole range of gynaecological ailments. In many western kitchens, the stems and seeds are used in confectionery and culinary flavourings. Its constituents are volatile oil, and bitter, astringent substances. It is warming and stimulating to the digestive system, lungs and circulation, and also carminative and expectorant to improve the body's ability to cope with cold.

The use of angelica goes back to antiquity and the root has been used since time immemorial to ward off poisons and epidemic diseases. Grown mainly in the provinces of Shanxi, Gansu, Sichuan and Yunnan in China, its main function in Chinese herbalism is to nourish the blood. Chinese herbalists recommend different parts of the root to address specific ailments.

The topmost part of the root, called *gui tou*, is used to stem bleeding. The tail end, *gui wei*, is used to enhance blood circulation, remove blood stagnation, alleviate pain, lubricate the intestines and prevent haemorrhage. The middle part, *gui shen,* is used for pregnancy problems especially for Qi circulation. In general health maintenance, the whole root is used. Whichever part is used, it is always sliced paper-thin.

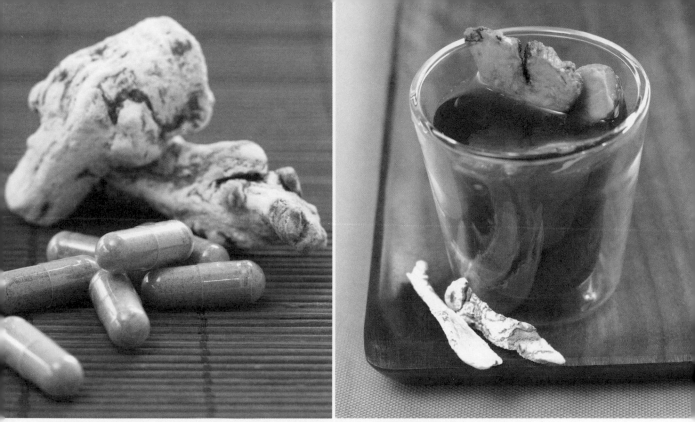

FROM LEFT TO RIGHT: Treatment: Chinese Angelica Pills for Nourishing Skin (page 37), Chinese Angelica Wine (page 37)

Chinese Angelica Wine

This tipple can become a woman's best friend without fear of being called a lush! It is excellent for alleviating menstrual pains and extremely warming for the soul when you are suffering from post-birth exhaustion.

Preparation time: 10 minutes
Serves 10–12

Chinese angelica slices 100 g (3¹/₂ oz)
Cognac 500 ml (16 fl oz / 2 cups)

Place Chinese angelica slices in a colander and rinse clean. Drain well, then pat dry with paper towels, making sure each slice is dry to the touch.

Place angelica slices in a clean glass bottle. Add cognac and leave to steep in a cool, dark place for up to 6 weeks.

Check that angelica slices are completely immersed as they can go mouldy otherwise.

Drink wine as required.

Treatments
Chinese angelica pills are an enriching herbal product because they often also contain treated foxglove root. When combined, the two herbs are said to nourish the skin from within and restore its natural, lustrous condition. The pills also help the body to rid itself of excess mucus and are effective in improving fat metabolism. Creams made from Chinese angelica are regenerating, and contain a natural oestrogen-like oil that helps to promote youthful and beautiful skin.

Aromatherapy
Chinese angelica tonic oil is a stimulating and refreshing unguent that helps to activate the flow of Qi and blood. When applied topically, it provides relief from sore or stiff necks and muscle pains.

Chinese chive

Common Chinese chive
Mandarin Jiu cai
Cantonese Gow choy
Botanical Allium tuberosum

A common enough herb, indispensable in mee siam and held to the bosom of most Chinese for its culinary versatility and medicinal promise, chives come in three forms. They are green with slim, flat leaves, yellow because they are grown with a cloche, or flowering with pale green buds. Crunchy aromatic taste aside, chives in Chinese herbalism are used for their warming and blood purifying properties, and also for the improvement of stomach, liver, kidney and skin functions. Chive seeds are purported to strengthen Yang energy and alleviate impotence.

Stir-fried Chinese Chives, Bean Curd and Salted Fish

Chinese chives are held to the bosom of every Chinese, especially those from the north. My neighbours, who are from Liaoning, rather than grow flowers and fruits, prefer to give over a large tract of their garden to growing them. I call it a vegetable with attitude. Now this is a truly rustic dish with peasant history, not for its simplicity but that it is a vegetable of the people. Served with plain congee, it does satisfy more than the appetite.

Preparation time: 10 minutes
Cooking time: 15 minutes
Serves 4

Vegetable oil 2 Tbsp

Salted threadfin (*ikan kurau*) 100 g (3¹/₂ oz)

Garlic 2 cloves, peeled and crushed

Chinese chives 80 g (3 oz), cut into 5-cm (2-in) lengths, then washed and drained

Bean sprouts 80 g (3 oz), washed and drained

Sesame oil 2 Tbsp

Heat oil in a wok or pan and fry salted fish over low heat until crisp and fragrant. Remove, cool and shred roughly.

In remaining oil, fry crushed garlic until golden brown, then throw in chives and bean sprouts and stir-fry over high heat for 2 minutes.

Add shredded salted fish and sesame oil and toss for 30 seconds more before dishing out to serve with plain congee and other dishes.

FROM LEFT TO RIGHT: Stir-fried Chinese Chives, Bean Curd and Salted Fish (page 39), Treatment: Poultice for Skin Rash (page 40)

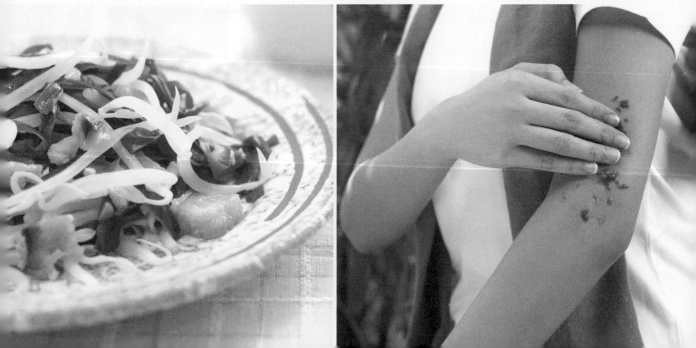

Chinese Chives with Pork Liver

This crunchy and succulent combination is deemed to be good for curing excessive perspiration and to stimulate sluggish appetites. The oyster sauce is my own take on giving this dish a well-rounded flavour.

Preparation time: 15 minutes
Cooking time: 10 minutes
Serves 4

Pig's liver 450 g (1 lb)

Chinese cooking wine (*shao hsing*) 2 Tbsp

Oyster sauce 1 Tbsp

Vegetable oil 2 Tbsp

Garlic 2 cloves, peeled and crushed

Chinese chives 80 g (3 oz), cut into 5-cm (2-in) lengths, washed and drained

Salt 1 tsp

Ground black pepper 1 tsp

Water 100 ml (3¹/₂ fl oz)

Wash and drain liver, then place in the freezer for about 20 minutes to firm up; this facilitates slicing it into thin pieces.

Combine liver slices, wine and oyster sauce in a bowl, then mix well and leave to marinate for 5 minutes.

Heat oil in a wok or pan and fry garlic for 1 minute, then add liver with its marinade, chives, salt and pepper. Stir-fry over high heat for 1 minute, then add water. Bring to a brisk boil for 2 minutes and remove from heat. Serve hot with rice and other dishes.

There is now in the market, a concentrated chive oil that works much like sesame oil in culinary usage and adds a fragrant top note to many dishes. A few drops of it in a stir-fry gives the finished dish a distinctive and delightful perfume.

Chive Wine

This is a potent drink to relieve minor internal injuries.

Chinese chives 50 g (2 oz)

Red wine 300 ml (10 fl oz)

Cut chives into small pieces and simmer them very gently in red wine for a few minutes.

Drink it warm.

Treatments

For the treatment of minor skin rash, apply a **poultice of ground chives** over the affected area for relief. The pure ground paste can also be applied directly to sunburn. Keep poultices on for 15–20 minutes before removing. To make a **chive milk for sore throat**, pound a small bunch of chives using a mortar and pestle, then strain and mix the juice with 250 ml (8 fl oz / 1 cup) milk and drink to soothe the throat.

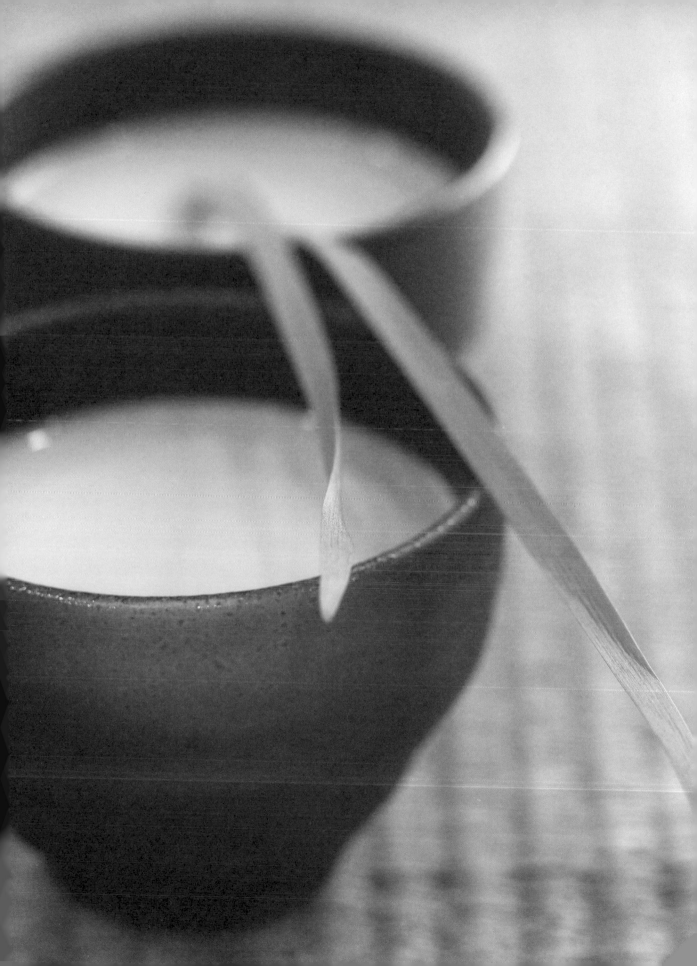

These dried wrinkly fruits, the size of grapes, are very different from the Mediterranean variety. Strictly speaking, the Chinese regard them as food first, but they do contain properties in restoring vigour and vitality. There are two main varieties, red and black, which are derived from two different treatments. When fresh dates are dried in the sun, they become red dates. Fresh dates that are boiled or steamed become black dates. Red dates are the preferred variety for food and herbal preparations as well as for drinks. A third variety, honeyed dates, known as *mi zao* in Mandarin or *mat choh* in Cantonese are sometimes used in sweet herbal drinks, obviating the need for sugar. However, they are more often consumed as a festive snack to symbolise a sweet life during the Chinese New Year.

Chicken with Red Dates, Ginger and Mushrooms

Mushrooms, especially shiitake, are not merely fungi in Chinese herbalism as they are known to combat certain cancers, lower blood cholesterol and help prevent rickets, anaemia and measles.

Preparation time: 15 minutes
Cooking time: 45 minutes
Serves 4

Dried or fresh shiitake mushrooms 10

Chicken 1 kg (2 lb 3 oz), cleaned and trimmed of excess fat

Chinese red dates 20, pitted, washed and drained

Fresh ginger 4 slices

Water 1 litre (32 fl oz / 4 cups)

Salt 2 tsp

Ground black pepper 1 tsp

If using dried mushrooms, soak them in hot water or boil them briefly until they are very soft. Cut away hard stems then halve each cap or leave whole, as desired. If using fresh mushrooms, simply wipe clean with paper towels before use.

Combine all ingredients in a pot and simmer for 45–60 minutes, depending on how tender you want your chicken. Serve hot with rice and other dishes.

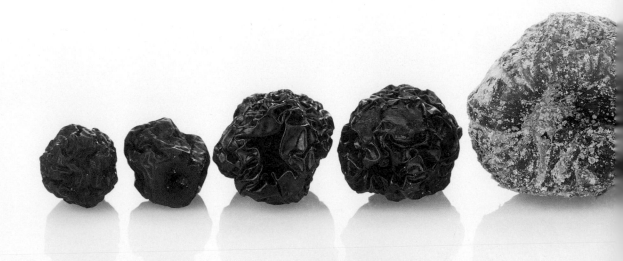

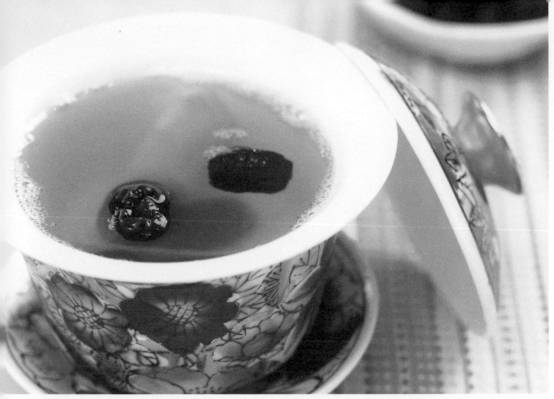

Ginger Tea with Honey and Red Dates (page 43)

Ginger Tea with Honey and Red Dates

This tea is excellent for alleviating 'cold' stomachs, abdominal pain and diarrhoea.

Preparation time: 10 minutes
Cooking time: 20 minutes
Serves 4

Water 600 ml (20 fl oz / 2½ cups)

Chinese red dates 60 g (2 oz), pitted, washed and drained

Fresh ginger 4 thin slices

Honey 2 Tbsp

Bring water to the boil in a pot. Add dates and ginger and simmer for 10 minutes. Switch off heat, cover pot and let steep for 10 minutes.

Add honey and stir to incorporate. Serve hot.

Common Chinese date

Mandarin Hong zao, Hei zao, Mi zao

Cantonese Hong choh, Hak choh, Mat choh

Botanical Ziziphus jujuba

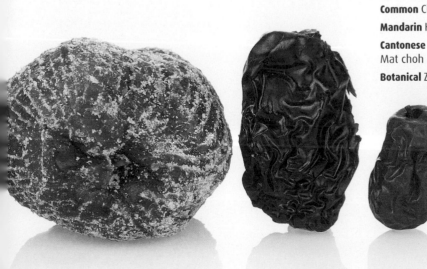

Chinese Wolfberry

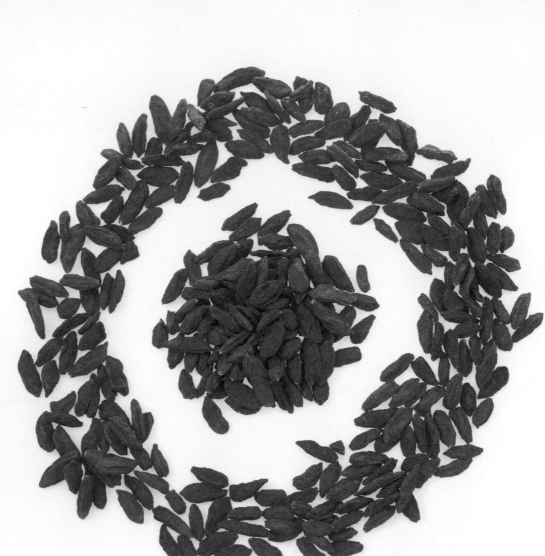

Common Chinese wolfberry
Mandarin Gou qi zi
Cantonese Gow gei chi
Botanical Lycium barbarum fructus

These small red seeds are from a plant found in East Asia and Inner Mongolia. Both the fruit and bark are used in medicine to improve vision and renal function. Wolfberries are believed to be remedial for diabetes, anaemia and chronic coughs. They also enrich Yin and 'lubricate' the lungs. Extremely palatable, the berries impart a sweetish flavour to most rich stews and soups.

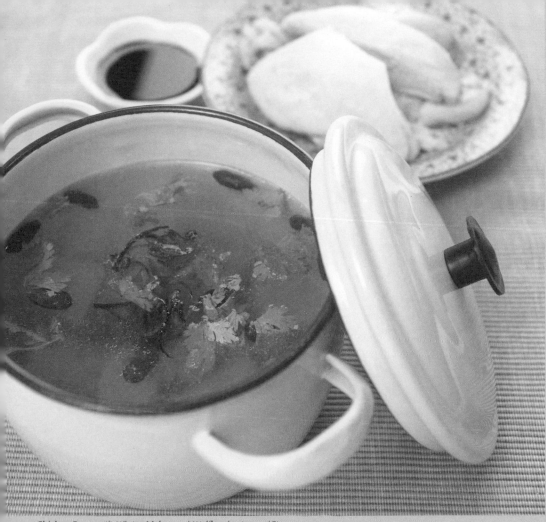

Chicken Soup with Winter Melon and Wolfberries (page 45)

Chicken Soup with Winter Melon and Wolfberries

There are any number of herbal dishes that use this sweet berry to good effect. Even children are given handfuls to munch to improve their eyesight. This is the simplest way of sweetening and enhancing the restorative elements of a chicken dish that is a soup as well as solid sustenance.

Preparation time: 15 minutes
Cooking time: 1 hour
Serves 4

Chicken 1.5 kg (3 lb 4 1/2 oz), cleaned and trimmed of excess fat

Chinese wolfberries 3 Tbsp, rinsed and drained

Water 1.5 litres (48 fl oz / 6 cups)

Salt 1 Tbsp

Ground black pepper 1 tsp

Winter melon 450 g (1 lb), peeled, pith removed and cut into chunks

Dark soy sauce to taste

Chopped fresh coriander leaves (cilantro) (optional)

Crisp-fried shallots (optional)

Either leave cleaned chicken whole, or cut into large joints. Combine chicken, wolfberries, water, salt and pepper in a pot. Simmer over medium heat for 30 minutes.

Add winter melon and simmer for 15 minutes. Serve soup first, garnished with chopped fresh coriander and a sprinkling of fried shallots, if desired.

Serve chicken joints afterwards, with a side dip of dark soy sauce. Most of the chicken's flavour would have gone into the soup with simmering, and the chicken will taste a little bland, hence the dip.

Note: If you are making this dish in advance, allow to cool completely before skimming fat off the surface for a less oily dish.

Chinese Yam

The plant from which these chalk-white slivers are produced, grow in Korea and in the provinces of Henan and Hunan in China. Also referred to as *huai shan* in Mandarin, which corresponds with its Cantonese name of *wai san*, it is named as such, as the Huaishan region in China is believed to produce the best of its kind.

Chinese yam has a sweetish, neutral flavour, with constituents that help to stabilise kidney, lung and spleen functions. It strengthens and improves digestion and supports respiration. The herb is often prescribed for treating diarrhoea, diabetes, wheezing, body weakness and urinary problems.

Common Chinese yam
Mandarin Shan yao, Huai shan
Cantonese Wai san
Botanical Dioscorea opposita radix

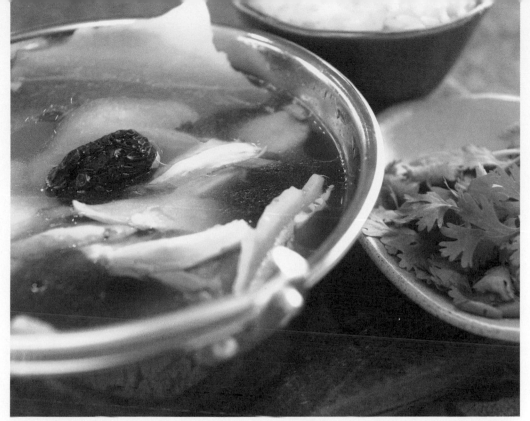

Chicken Soup with Chinese Yam, Chinese Angelica and Black Dates (page 47)

Chicken Soup with Chinese Yam, Chinese Angelica and Black Dates

This is a powerhouse of a soup that nourishes the blood and strengthens Qi. Traditionally, it is slow-cooked for up to 6 hours and then only the soup is drunk; the chicken being discarded. You do not have to be a stickler for tradition, and cooking this in a pressure cooker will do as well. And eat the chicken as well, albeit most of the flavour has gone into the soup.

Preparation time: 15 minutes
Cooking time: 1 hour 30 minutes or 45 minutes (pressure cooker)
Serves 4

Chicken 1, about 1.5 kg (3 lbs 4 1/2 oz), cleaned and trimmed of excess fat

Dried Chinese yam slices 20 g (2/3 oz)

Chinese angelica 10 g (1/3 oz)

Black dates 10, pitted, rinsed and drained

Sesame oil 2 Tbsp

Salt 2 tsp

Sugar 1 tsp

Ground black pepper 1 tsp

Fresh ginger slices 20 g (2/3 oz)

Chinese cooking wine (*shao hsing*) 3 Tbsp

Water 1.5 litres (48 fl oz / 6 cups)

Spring onions (scallions) 2 stalks, chopped

Fresh coriander (cilantro) 1 bunch, coarsely chopped

Combine all ingredients except spring onions and coriander in a deep pot.

Cover, bring to the boil and simmer for 1 hour 30 minutes, or until chicken is fork-tender. If you are using a pressure cooker, reduce water to 1 litre and pressure cook for 40–45 minutes.

To serve, remove skin and bones from chicken and shred meat coarsely. Return meat to soup. Serve with chopped spring onions and coriander on the side for diners to help themselves, and accompany with rice if desired.

Note: If you prefer to have a low-fat soup, remove all skin from the chicken. However, the flavour of the soup will not be as rich.

Potstickers with Chinese Yam

Preparation time: 15 minutes
Cooking time: 45 minutes
Serves 4

Minced pork or chicken 140 g (5 oz)

Finely grated, peeled fresh Chinese yam 4 Tbsp

Cornflour (cornstarch) 2 Tbsp

Chopped Chinese chives 3 Tbsp

Sesame oil 2 Tbsp

Salt 2 tsp

Sugar 1 tsp

Ground black pepper 1 tsp

Round potsticker skins 20–30

Water 125 ml (4 fl oz / $^1/_2$ cup)

Cooking oil

Side Dip

Chinese black vinegar 4 Tbsp

Shredded young ginger 1 Tbsp

Sugar $^1/_2$ tsp

Light soy sauce $^1/_2$ tsp

Prepare side dip. Combine ingredients together and set aside.

Prepare potstickers. Combine all ingredients except potsticker skins, water and cooking oil. Mix well and check for seasoning.

Lay a round skin on a clean work surface. Place a scant teaspoon of filling in the skin's centre. Brush rim of skin lightly with water. Fold skin in half. Pinch the apex of the semicircle to seal, then make small pleats in the skin edge nearest to you, on each side of the central pinch. (The skin edge away from you remains unpleated.) Press pleats to seal. The result should be a compact dumpling with a lightly curved sealed top edge (see picture on page 49).

Heat a well-seasoned frying pan with a little oil over medium heat. Arrange dumplings in pan. Fry in batches if necessary, and cook for 2–3 minutes, or until their bottoms are lightly browned.

Pour water into pan and cover. Cook for about 2 minutes, or until almost all the water has evaporated. Uncover and cook for another 2–3 minutes, until pan is dry and dumplings are well-browned on the bottom. Drizzle a little more oil into the pan to help them brown, if necessary.

Serve hot as a snack with side dip, adjusting amount of side dip as desired.

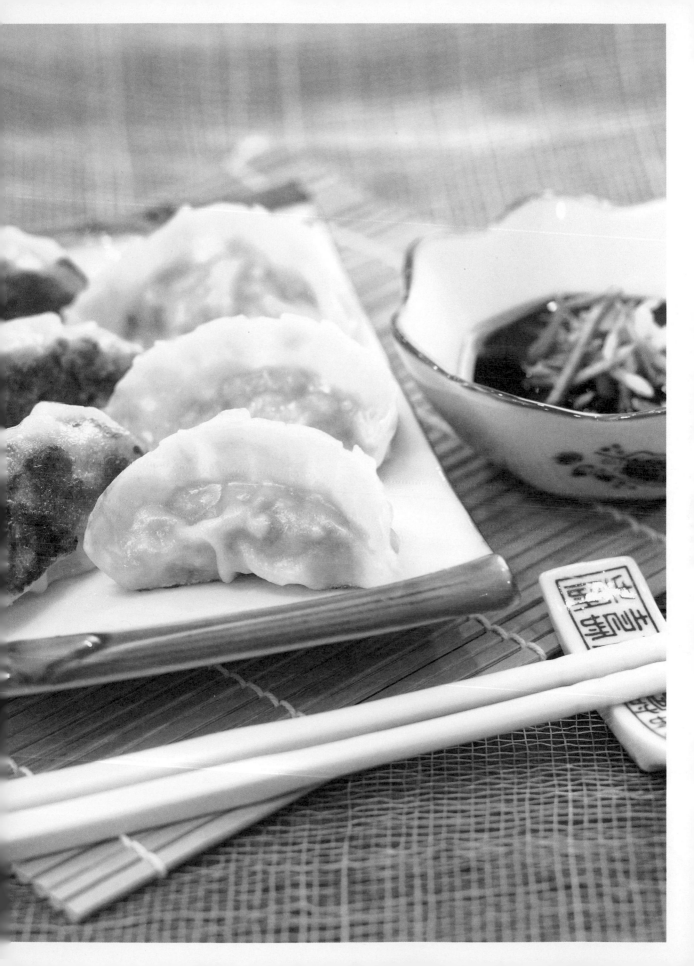

Chrysanthemum

Common Chrysanthemum
Mandarin Ju hua
Cantonese Kohk fah
Botanical Chrysanthemum morifolium flos

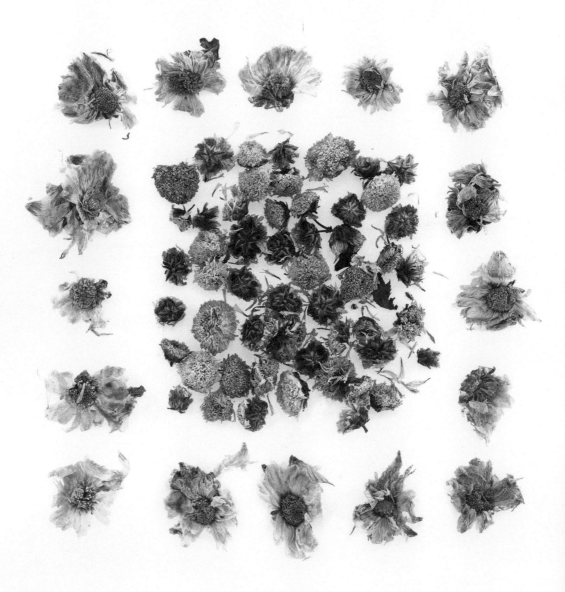

Infusing flower petals in hot water to extract fragrance is by no means an exclusive Chinese practice. Early Europeans were imbibing chamomile, magnolia and camellia tea long before Earl Grey graced the inner sanctums of every English drawing room. But it was the Chinese who made an art of brewing all manner of drinks from magnolia, chrysanthemum and other more obscure blooms.

Perhaps more than any other blossom, the chrysanthemum is held with absolute reverence for its efficacy in a whole host of ailments. These range from a weak liver, poor eyesight, bad blood circulation, infections and digestive upsets to nervous disorders, menstrual irregularity, graying hair and unhealthy blood. Indeed, there was an age-old Chinese belief that if you drank from a stream that flowed between the chrysanthemum blooms, you would live for 100 years. Even the dew from the leaves were purported to promote good health. In China, the Chong Jiu Double Ninth festival held on the 9th day of the 9th Lunar Month, was a time for the ceremonial drinking of chrysanthemum wine, and coincided with vast displays of the blooms.

In food and herbal preparations, the two most commonly used species are the *chrysanthemum indicum,* which grows wild in most parts of China except the cold north, and *chrysanthemum morifolium,* commonly cultivated in pots in Singapore, other parts of Southeast Asia, and in the Chinese provinces of Anhui and Zhejiang. The leaf of the variety called 'garland chrysanthemum' is known as *tung hao* in Mandarin or *tong ho* in Cantonese. It is a featured vegetable in steamboat meals.

Chrysanthemum and Wolfberry Tea (page 52)

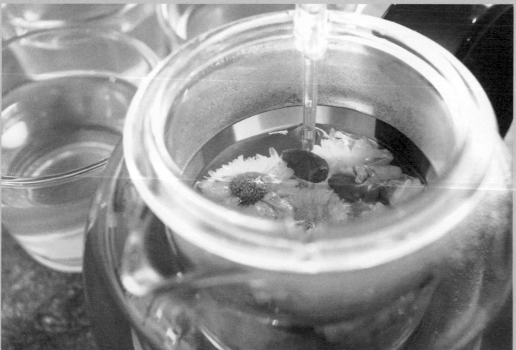

Chrysanthemum and Wolfberry Tea

This blend soothes the heart, removes liver heat and regulates the blood pressure. It is best drunk after a surfeit of rich food. The wolfberries are sweet and obviate the need to add sugar, but you can add a little rock sugar if you have a sweet tooth.

Preparation time: 10 minutes
Cooking time: 15 minutes
Serves 4

Water 1 litre (32 fl oz / 4 cups)

Rock sugar (optional) 20 g ($^2/_3$ oz)

Chinese wolfberries 10 g ($^1/_3$ oz), rinsed and drained

Dried chrysanthemum flowers 10 g ($^1/_3$ oz), rinsed and drained

Bring water to the boil with rock sugar, if using. Add remaining ingredients and let steep for 15 minutes.

Strain and serve warm.

Chrysanthemum Chicken Salad

I was shown how to combine these blooms with chicken by the late venerable doyen of Chinese cookery, Kenneth Lo. Rather like using nasturtium flowers in a salad, there is a certain culinary éclat to it. The fact is that the Chinese have revered and used chrysanthemum flowers as a food for centuries, as much for culinary reasons as for longevity and dissolving spiritual blockages.

Preparation time: 15 minutes
Cooking time: 15 minutes
Serves 4

Chicken breast 450 g (1 lb)

Cucumber $^1/_2$, peeled and shredded

Sweet mango 1, peeled, seeded and julienned

Dried chrysanthemum flowers 10 g ($^1/_3$ oz), rinsed, drained and dried on paper towels

Dressing (combined)

Olive oil 2 Tbsp

Wine vinegar 1 Tbsp

Salt 1 tsp

Sugar 1 tsp

Bring a small pot of water to the boil, add chicken and simmer for 10 minutes, or until cooked. Cool and shred.

Toss chicken with cucumber and mango in a mixing bowl. Drizzle dressing all over and toss a few times more to mix, then transfer to a serving plate.

Dot salad with chrysanthemum flowers. For good measure, decorate with a few fresh chrysanthemums, if available. Refrigerate for a while and serve chilled.

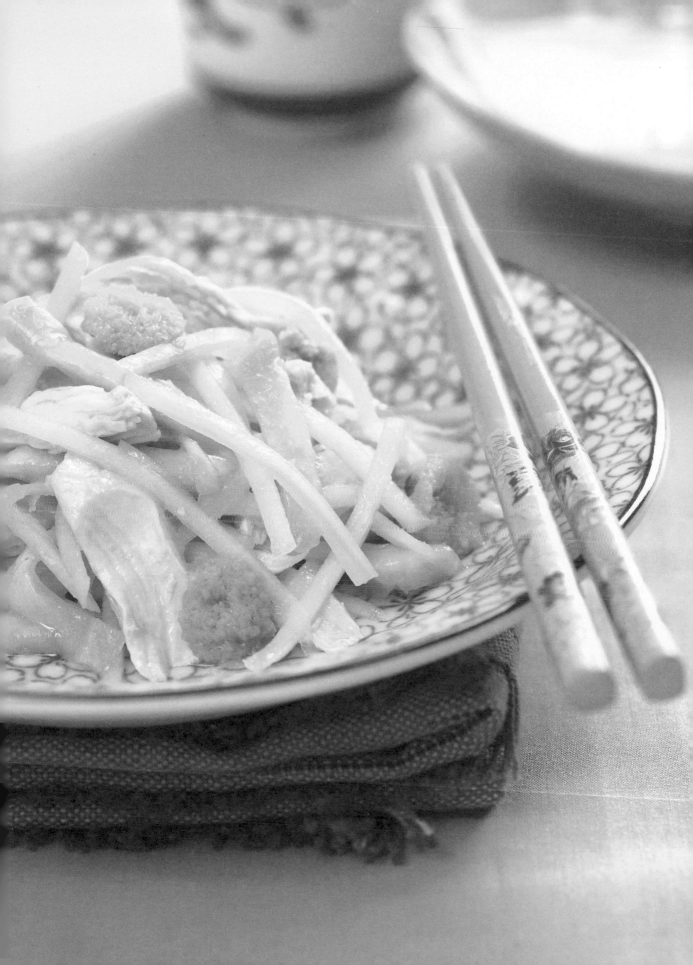

Cinnamon

A member of the cassia family, the cinnamon tree is grown widely in the Himalayas, Sri Lanka, China and Southeast Asia.

The most common herbal type is the bark of the Chinese cinnamon known as *rou gui*, which is thick, rich in oils and has a deep brown colour. A warm and pungent ingredient with constituents of volatile oil, tannins, mucilage and sugars, cinnamon is taken to warm the heart and bladder channels, dispel cold and activate blood and Qi circulation. It is also commonly used to treat colds, profuse sweating, painful joints and menstrual and heart problems. Cinnamon essential oil is a potent anti-bacterial and anti-fungal agent, as well as a uterine stimulant.

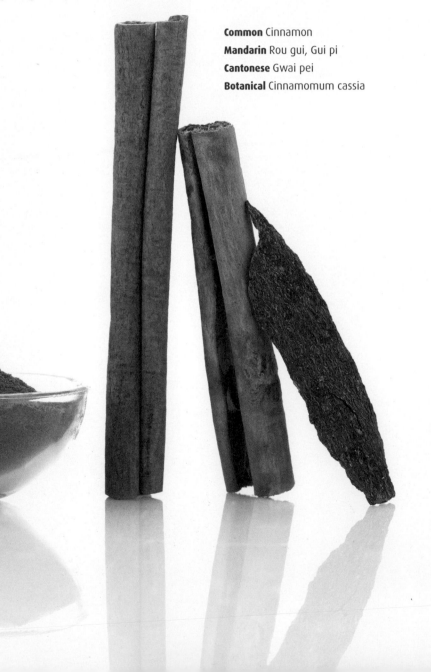

Common Cinnamon
Mandarin Rou gui, Gui pi
Cantonese Gwai pei
Botanical Cinnamomum cassia

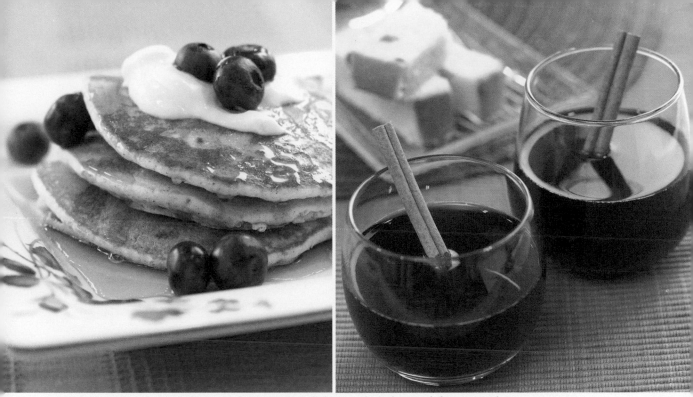

FROM LEFT TO RIGHT: Cinnamon and Blueberry Pancakes (page 55), Mulled Wine with Cinnamon and Cloves (page 56)

Cinnamon and Blueberry Pancakes

I am very partial to blueberries, especially in muffins and pancakes. This is a very beguiling recipe, and one that I was served on a blueberry farm in Canada. It is guaranteed to win you fans.

Preparation time: 25 minutes
Cooking time: 15 minutes
Serves 4

Plain (all-purpose) flour 200 g (7 oz)

Caster (superfine)sugar 100 g (3¹/₂ oz)

Baking powder 1 tsp

Ground cinnamon ¹/₂ tsp

Salt a pinch

Egg 1

Semi-skimmed milk 250 ml (8 fl oz / 1 cup)

Vegetable or corn oil 2 Tbsp

Topping

Fresh or canned blueberries 280 g (10 oz)

Fresh single cream

Maple syrup (optional)

Sift flour into a mixing bowl and mix with sugar, baking powder, cinnamon and salt.

Whisk egg with milk in a separate bowl, then blend with flour mixture. Stir until smooth and lump-free.

Heat oil in a pan and add a ladleful each time to fry into a pancake. Flip over when underside is light brown. When the other side is also light brown, remove and keep warm, covered with paper towels, as you finish cooking.

Serve 1 or 2 pancakes with a generous tablespoonful of blueberries, a good dollop of fresh cream and drizzle all over with maple syrup, if desired.

Mulled Wine with Cinnamon and Cloves

I was once served this delicious concoction during the Christmas season by a Jewish lady, one of my cookery students. To my comment that 'Jewish people do not celebrate Christmas', she countered, 'I am not celebrating Christmas, I am celebrating mulled wine!' Touché.

Preparation time: 15 minutes
Cooking time: 10 minutes
Serves 4–6

Claret (dry red wine) 600 ml
(20 fl oz / 2 ½ cups)

Cloves 4

Orange 1, small

Brown sugar 2 Tbsp

Cinnamon 2 sticks,
10-cm (4-in) long each

Pour wine into a clean glass or enamel container with a mouth large enough to accommodate orange.

Poke cloves into the rind of orange, then add to wine to steep. Cover container and leave to macerate for 24 hours.

Remove orange and pour wine into a clean pan. Bring to a gentle boil, then add sugar and cinnamon. Remove from heat.

Leave to steep for 4–5 hours, then remove cinnamon. Heat wine to a gentle warmth and serve in mugs. It is all icky, sticky and marvellous, served with cinnamon pancakes.

Treatments

There are proprietary tablets that contain cinnamon which are taken to help clear eye conditions and lower blood pressure. Cinnamon is said to improve fat metabolism and gently relieve constipation.

Aromatherapy

Cinnamon essential oil is extracted from the leaves of the plant and is usually used in a blend for its heady scent. Ideally blended with orange or nutmeg oil, it becomes an excellent vaporiser that helps to clear the air of any musty smell with its spicy-sweet aroma. When placed in a burner, or in the oil for garden torches, it helps to dispel insects.

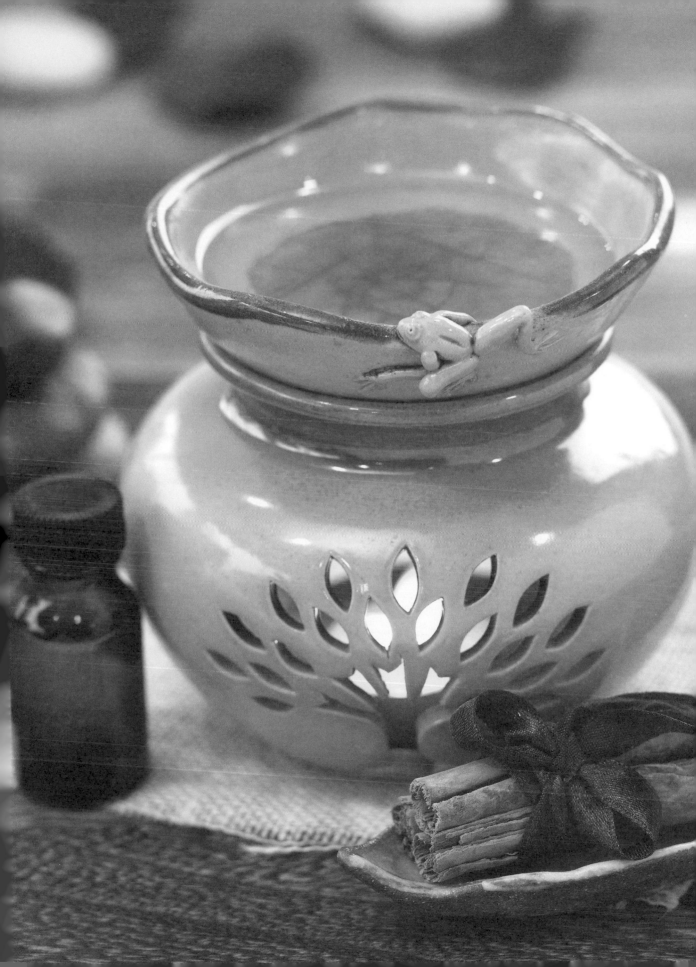

Clove

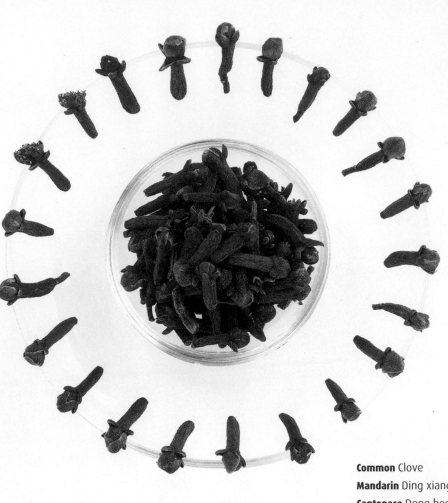

Common Clove
Mandarin Ding xiang
Cantonese Deng heong
Botanical Syzygium aromaticum,
Eugenia caryophyllata

Of the family *myrtaceae*, the spice has been known worldwide since the 5th century. In India, cloves are chewed with betel leaves as a digestive aid, and are still used in Greek medicinal formulations today. Though primarily used as a culinary herb by the Chinese, the oil extracted from the dried flower buds of the plant has carminative and stimulating actions. Its warm constituents influence the kidney, spleen and stomach channels, as well as alleviate Qi and regulate blood circulation. The spice also aids digestion, reduces wind, and soothes toothache and colic. Its astringent qualities are good for removing toxins from the body. A paste of ground cloves, when applied externally, is good for the treatment of insect bites, cuts and swelling.

Tiffin Pork Chops

I believe this is a colonial invention (hence the inclusion of Worcestershire sauce here), and one that sits squarely within the Singapore culinary genre, turning up at such august places as the Raffles Hotel, and way down the social scale, at cheap and cheerful *kopi tiams*.

Preparation time: 20 minutes
Cooking time: 25 minutes
Serves 4–6

Pork chops 2, each about 2-cm (1-in) thick

Egg 1, beaten

Cream crackers 10, crushed finely

Cooking oil for shallow frying

Potatoes 2, peeled and cut into 0.5-cm (¼-in) thick slices

Tomatoes 2, halved and sliced thickly

Sauce (combined)

Dark soy sauce 2 Tbsp

Worcestershire sauce 2 Tbsp

Sugar 1 Tbsp

Cloves 6

Light soy sauce 1 tsp

Black pepper 1 tsp

Water 400 ml (13 fl oz / 1¾ cups)

With a sharp knife, butterfly pork chops and open out flat, to obtain 2 thin escalopes. Tenderise escalopes briefly with a meat mallet or the back of a cleaver, then wash and drain. Dip escalopes in beaten egg, turning to coat thoroughly, then dredge with cracker crumbs. Press crumbs firmly onto meat to get a thin, even coating. Set aside for 15 minutes in the fridge, covered, to firm up.

Heat oil in a pan and fry potatoes for 3–4 minutes, or until half-cooked and light brown. Remove and set aside to drain on paper towels.

Fry pork escalopes in oil until golden brown, then drain well. Let cool for 10 minutes, then chop into bite-sized pieces.

Pour combined sauce ingredients into a wok and bring to the boil. Add potatoes and cook for 2 minutes over high heat, until sauce has reduced by one-third. Add tomatoes and simmer for 1 minute, or until sauce is thick and glossy. Remove and discard cloves.

Add sliced pork chops to the pan and toss to mix. Remove from heat and serve immediately with rice or bread.

Treatments

Clove oil is well-known as a pain-killer for toothaches. An **orange studded with cloves** not only gives off a lovely perfume, but also acts as a natural insect repellent.

Aromatherapy

Like its spicy sister, cinnamon, **clove essential oil** is also an extract from the leaves of the parent plant. It is most frequently used as an insect repellent, and as an ingredient in mothballs. It is a warm, sweet and spicy oil for aromatherapy burners when blended with other citrus oils like orange or citronella. Not recommended for massage.

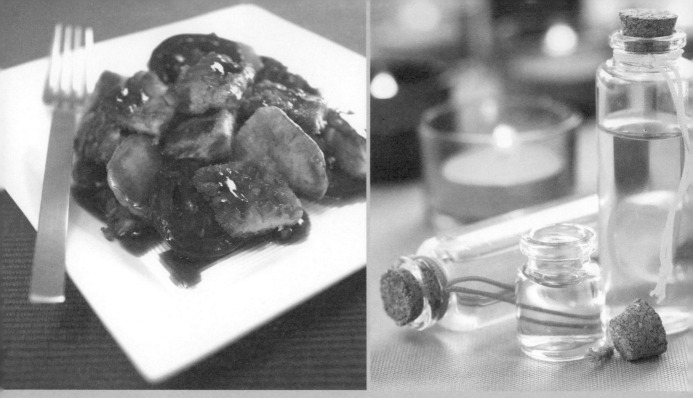

FROM LEFT TO RIGHT: *Tiffin Pork Chops (page 59), Aromatherapy: Clove Essential Oil (page 59), Treatment: Natural Insect Repellent (page 59)*

Spicy Chicken and Clove Soup

Many moons ago, my father, who hailed from Indonesia, used to cook this soup that I still trot out every so often. It is aromatic, heady and very good for clearing a hangover.

Preparation time: 15 minutes
Cooking time: 25 minutes
Serves 4

Water 1 litre (32 fl oz / 4 cups)

Chicken thigh meat 150 g (5 oz)

Cloves 8

Celery 1 stalk, sliced

Shallots 5, peeled and sliced

Garlic 4 cloves, peeled and crushed

Red chillies 2, chopped

Ground black pepper 1 tsp

Chicken stock cube 1

Garnishing

Chopped spring onions (scallions) 2 Tbsp

Chopped mint 1 Tbsp

Bring water to the boil and cook all ingredients, except garnishing, for 15 minutes. Remove chicken to cool and continue to simmer soup for 10 minutes.

Meanwhile, shred chicken and set aside. Strain soup through a fine sieve to get a clear consommé.

Add chicken to soup and serve, garnished with spring onions and mint.

Note: You can add a handful of mung (green) bean vermicelli (tang hoon) that has been blanched in boiling water and drained, to each bowl of soup for extra oomph.

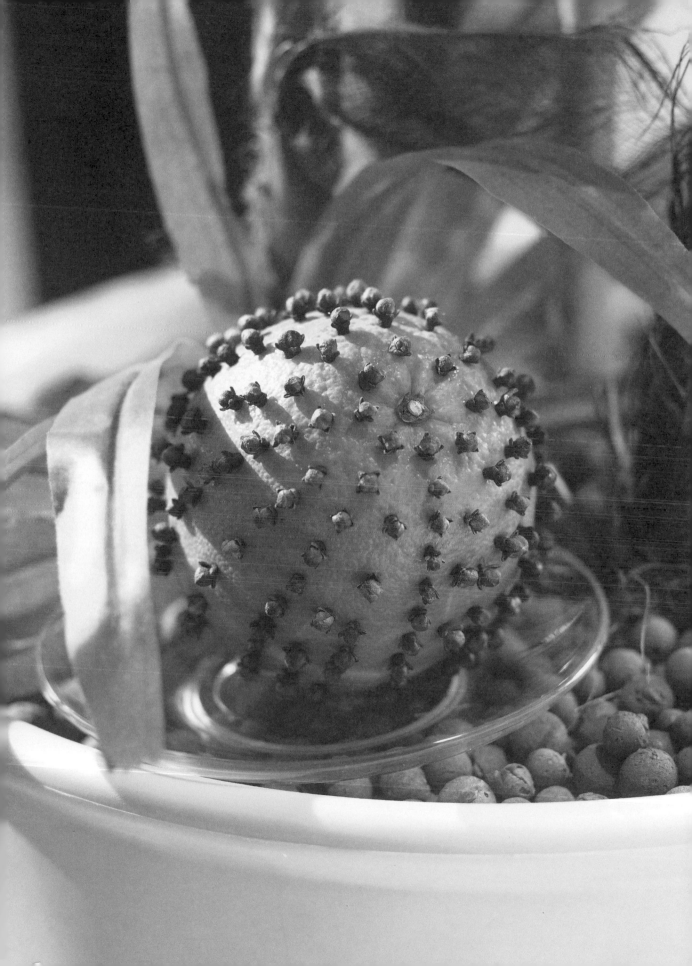

Codonopsis Root

Common Codonopsis root
Mandarin Dang shen
Cantonese Dong sam
Botanical Codonopsis pilosula radix

Two species of the root exist — one is a native of the region consisting of the former Manchuria and northern China, namely, the provinces of Inner Mongolia and Qinghai, while the other originates from Qinghai but has come to be cultivated in the central Chinese provinces of Sichuan and Hubei.

The root is generally used as a tonic and stimulant, reputedly good for the treatment of gonorrhea and gynaecological diseases, as well as regulating blood circulation. In some parts of Asia, it is widely adopted as a respectable substitute for the more expensive ginseng. Herbal medicine researchers have recorded that the extract of the codonopsis root can increase the number of red corpuscles and reduce the number of leucocytes in the blood. The codonopsis root is sometimes mistakenly identified as the mid-section of ginseng.

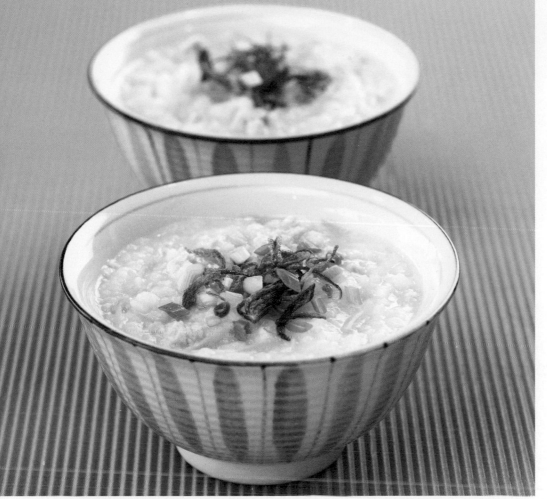

Congee with Minced Pork, Dried Scallops and Codonopsis Root (page 63)

Congee with Minced Pork, Dried Scallops and Codonopsis Root

The Cantonese are inordinately fond of cooking congee with dried scallops that, during the Chinese New Year season, can be horrendously expensive. However, a little goes a long way. This congee with codonopsis is hearty and curative enough to merit the spending of some greenbacks on the scallops. Broken rice gives a really smooth congee.

Preparation time: 20 minutes
Cooking time: 1 hour
Serves 4

Codonopsis root 10 g (¹/₃ oz), rinsed and drained

Water 2 litres (64 fl oz / 8 cups)

Dried scallops (*gan bei / kong yu chi*) 6

Broken rice 200 g (7 oz), washed and drained

Minced pork 150 g (5 oz)

Sesame oil 2 Tbsp

Salt 2 tsp

Ground black pepper 1 tsp

Fried shallots (optional)

Chopped spring onions (scallions) (optional)

Place codonopsis root and water in a large pot and boil for 25 minutes. Remove codonopsis and discard.

Add scallops and rice to herbal stock and return to the boil. Cook for 20 minutes or until rice is thick.

Add minced pork, sesame oil, salt and pepper and simmer for 15 minutes more. Serve hot, garnished with fried shallots and chopped spring onions, if desired.

Cordyceps

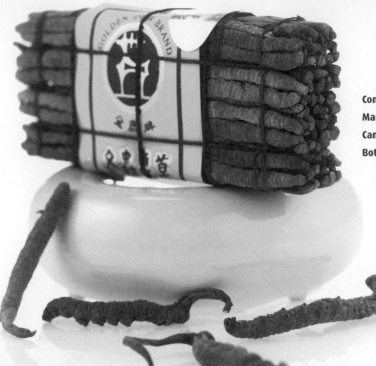

Common Cordyceps
Mandarin Dong chong xia cao
Cantonese Dong chong cho
Botanical Allium tuberosum

The Chinese name of the herb, *dong chong xia cao*, literally means 'winter worm summer grass'. It is likened to a lowly worm which creeps about in winter, undergoes a metamorphosis through spring to become a leaf in summer, dries up in autumn to drop like a shrivelled twig and begins its creepy-crawly cycle all over again. This strange herb is found mainly in the provinces of Sichuan, Qinghai, Guizhou and Yunnan in China and only experts, with the well-honed powers of truffle hunters, can pinpoint the exact underground lair of hibernation.

It certainly looks like a mummified creepy crawly with tiny, black, beady eyes that apparently fill with life when the cordycep is put to the boil. True to the Yin Yang philosophy of perfect balance and physical diagnosis based on elements of harmonious interaction, cordyceps are believed to rejuvenate and restore life's forces by virtue of its incredible ability for self-restoration.

As an ingredient reputedly vital to one's physical well-being, the cordycep has been cropping up frequently in various forms. You read about its efficacy in ginseng essence on advertisements posted on the back of buses, and in posters promoting herbal mixes hung above Chinese medicinal shop fronts. Chinese herbalists get positively persuasive, endorsing the herb's properties for improving vigour, impotence, lumbago and general debility.

Chicken Soup with Cordyceps

In the past decade, cordyceps have made a frequent appearance, most noticeably in commercially prepared ginseng essence and other chicken extracts. This is a soup that all mothers love to serve their children.

Preparation time: 15 minutes
Cooking time: 1 hour
Serves 4

Chicken 900 g (2 lb), cleaned and skinned

Cordyceps 30 g (1 oz), rinsed and drained

Water 1.5 litres (48 fl oz / 6 cups)

Salt 2 tsp

Combine all ingredients in a pot and simmer over very low heat for at least 1 hour.

Before serving, skim off as much fat as possible, and remove cordyceps. Debone chicken if desired, and serve with soup.

Duck Soup with Cordyceps

I am partial to duck and, having total faith in cordyceps, this is a soup I cook often.

Preparation time: 20 minutes
Cooking time: 2–3 hours or 1 hour (pressure cooker)
Serves 4

Water 2.5 litres (80 fl oz / 10 cups)

Duck 1, cleaned, skinned and cut into 8 joints

Cordyceps 20 g (²/₃ oz)

Preserved limes 2

Light soy sauce 2 Tbsp

Cognac or brandy 2 Tbsp

Bring water to the boil in a large pot. Add duck and cordyceps. Simmer, covered, for 1 hour 30 minutes.

Add limes and soy sauce and continue to cook for another 1 hour 30 minutes, or until duck meat falls off the bones.

Remove cordyceps and add cognac or brandy before serving.

Chicken Soup with Cordyceps (page 65)

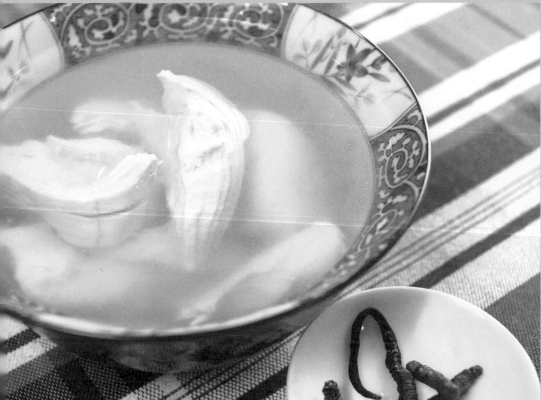

Coriander

Widely used by people in the Mediterranean region and Asia for centuries, both as a culinary herb, and for the treatment of ailments including indigestion, flatulence and colic, the coriander is, first of all, a very fragrant plant. Today, it is an essential herb in India, China, the Middle East and South America. A sprig of fresh coriander, when chopped and added to a soup or stew exudes a delicious perfume. In many Asian countries, coriander seeds are ground into powder and used as a key ingredient in curries. For medicinal purposes, the seeds, which contain volatile oils and tannin, have aromatic, carminative and stimulant actions; they can be coarsely ground and brewed into a tea for aiding digestion and warding off colds.

Coriander essential oil is believed to help improve memory when applied in aromatherapy. When taken internally, the oil can relieve asthma and rheumatism as well as detoxify the body and stimulate the spleen. It also aids in restoring hormonal balance in females and relieving menstrual cramps.

Common Coriander
Mandarin Yan sui
Cantonese Yeen sai
Botanical Coriandrum sativum

Herb Salad (page 68)

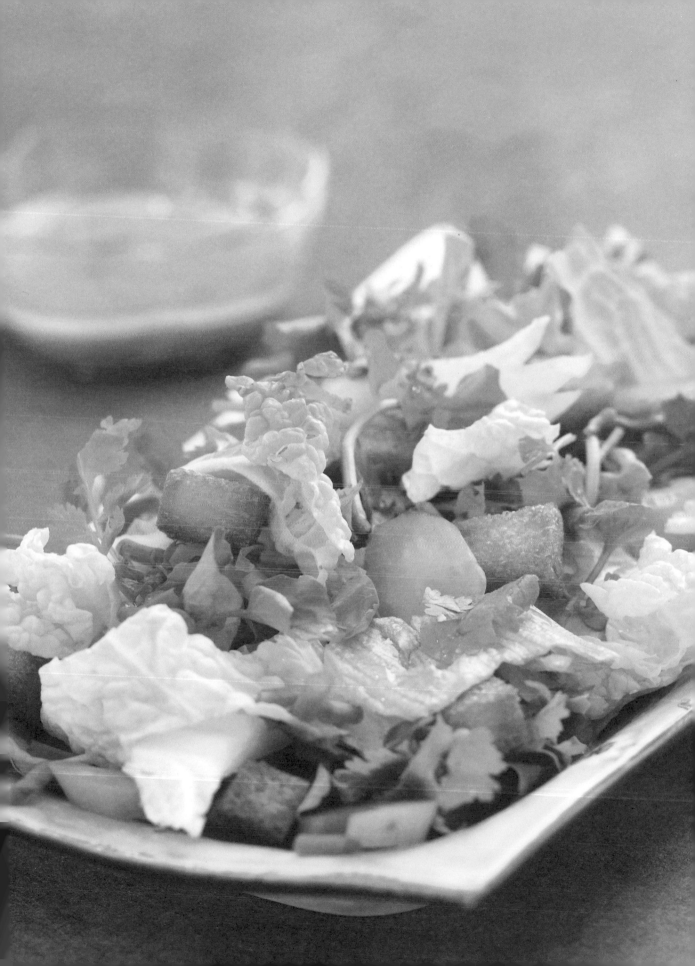

Herb Salad

This is a refreshing compendium of fresh green herbs that one rarely tires of. Really a seasonal dish, use whatever greens that are most topical and freshest.

Preparation time: 20 minutes
Serves 4–6

Watercress 60 g (2 oz)

Iceberg lettuce 60 g (2 oz)

Shanghai greens (*bok choy*) 60 g (2 oz)

Celery 60 g (2 oz)

Spring onions (scallions) 30 g (1 oz)

Coriander (cilantro) leaves 40 g (1^1/$_2$ oz)

Garlic croutons for garnish

Dressing

Lime juice 2 Tbsp

Yellow mustard 1 Tbsp

Rice wine 1 Tbsp

Sugar 1 Tbsp

Olive oil 2 Tbsp

Wash and dry all greens well. Cut up watercress roughly, shred lettuce into small pieces and slice bok choy into 2-cm (1-in) wide strips.

Slice celery into 1-cm (^{1}/$_2$-in) pieces diagonally. Chop spring onions and coriander leaves.

Place all cut greens in a salad bowl. Put dressing ingredients into a glass bottle, then cap and shake well.

Just before serving, pour dressing over salad and toss well. Garnish with croutons.

Smoked Salmon with Coriander Sauce

The aromatic zest of ground coriander roots, stem and leaves make a perfect foil for salty smoked salmon in this an appetising starter.

Preparation time: 10 minutes
Cooking time: 1 minute
Serves 4

Coriander (cilantro) 80 g (3 oz), with roots intact, washed and drained

Olive oil 2 Tbsp

Garlic 2 cloves, peeled

Salt ^{1}/$_2$ tsp

Lime juice 2 Tbsp

Smoked salmon 340 g (11^1/$_2$ oz)

Lemon 4 wedges

Combine coriander, olive oil, garlic and salt in a blender (processor), or spice grinder and blend until creamy.

Transfer purée to a microwavable bowl and blend in lime juice, then heat in a microwave oven for 1 minute on medium. Let cool, then refrigerate for 1 hour.

To serve, arrange slices of smoked salmon on serving plates and spoon coriander sauce over. Serve as an appetiser.

Treatments

A drink made by boiling 45 g (1^1/$_2$ oz) coriander leaves with 250 ml (8 fl oz/1 cup) water for 5 minutes, and taken warm, is believed to relieve symptoms associated with measles, especially if they have not developed fully.

To make a **drink for indigestion**, boil 1 tsp coriander seeds with a few pieces of dried orange peel and a large knob of peeled ginger in 250 ml (8 fl oz/1 cup) water for 5 minutes. Drink warm.

Aromatherapy

Coriander essential oil is derived from the seeds and is a strong stimulant. When blended with a base oil to use as a massage oil, it has an uplifting effect and dissipates fatigue. When combined on a burner, it gives off a pleasantly sweet, spicy and woody aroma of a provocative nature, that stokes a tired mind into action.

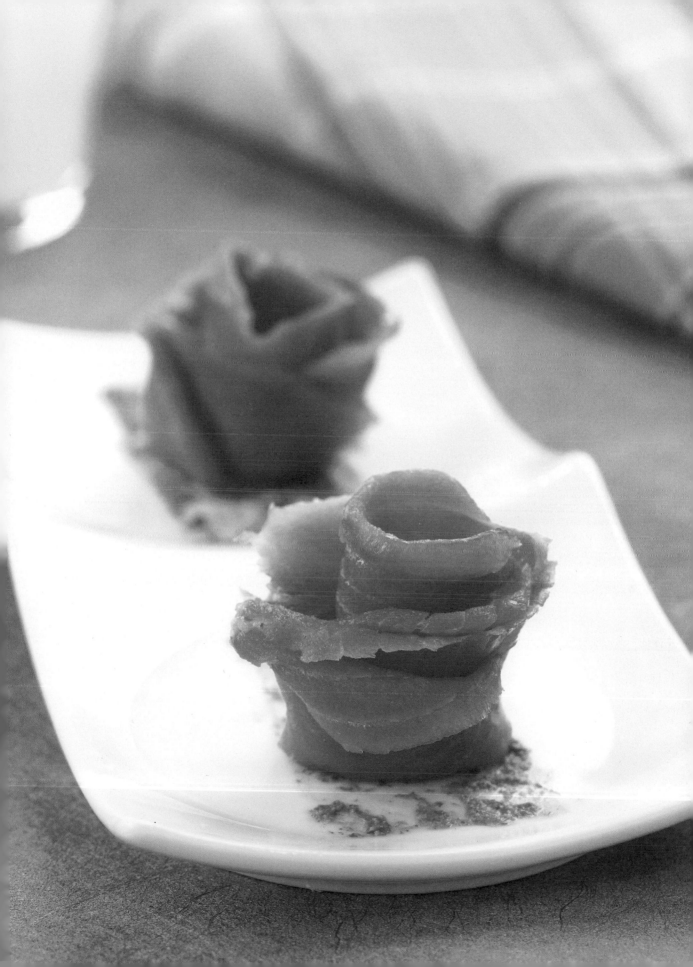

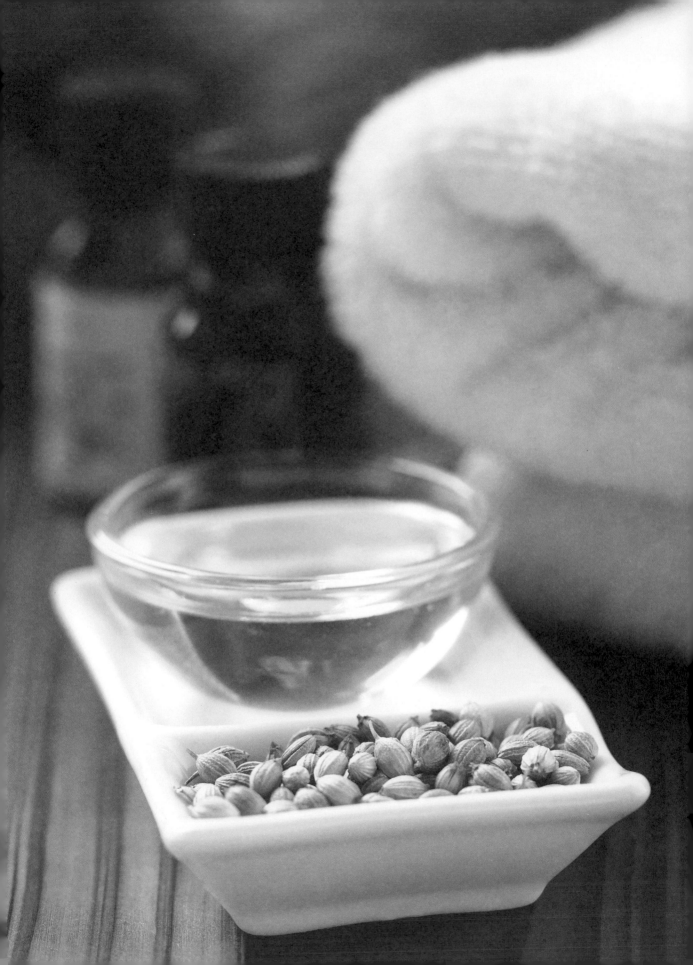

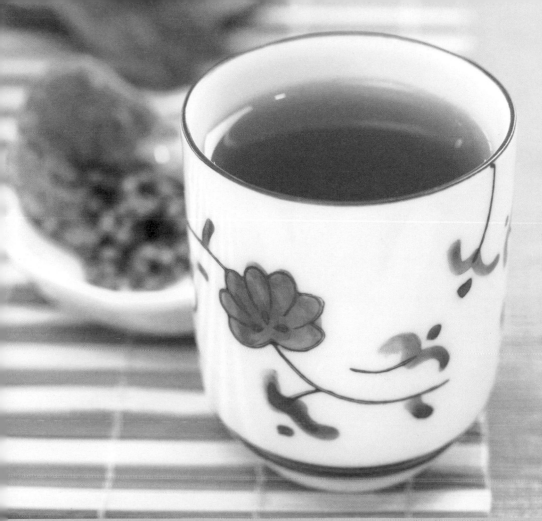

FROM LEFT TO RIGHT: Aromatherapy. Coriander Essential Oil (page 68), Treatment: Drink for Indigestion (page 68)

Coriander and Lemon Grass Chicken Stir-fry

This is a good Thai-Chinese standby that is easy and quick to prepare. Serve it with steamed coconut rice.

Preparation time: 15 minutes
Cooking time: 10 minutes
Serves 4

Cooking oil 2 Tbsp

Garlic 2 cloves, peeled and thinly sliced

Lemon grass 2, use lower 5 cm (2 in) only, thinly sliced

Chicken thigh meat 250 g (9 oz), cut into strips

Red chillies 2, sliced

Coriander (cilantro) 50 g (2 oz), washed, roots discarded and cut into 2.5-cm (1-in) lengths

Fish sauce 1 Tbsp

Sugar 1 tsp

Water 100 ml (3^{1}/$_{2}$ fl oz)

Cornflour (cornstarch) 1 Tbsp, mixed with 2 Tbsp water

Heat oil in a wok or pan and fry garlic and lemon grass for 2 minutes.

Add chicken, chillies and coriander and fry for 3 minutes. Season with fish sauce and sugar.

Add water and bring to a quick boil. Add cornflour mixture and stir until thickened. Serve hot with rice.

Cumin

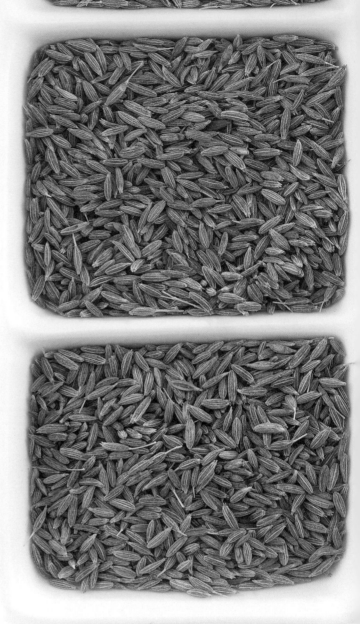

Common Cumin
Mandarin Zi ran
Cantonese
Botanical Cuminum cyminum

Indigenous to the Middle East, cumin was used during the time of the Pharaohs not only as a food spice, but also as a natural preservative to mummify deceased kings. From there, it was introduced to Greece and Rome, where the spice was used both as a medicine and as a cosmetic to induce a pale complexion. It appeared that students in ancient Greece and Rome would drink large quantities of cumin oil to induce a pallid complexion that was regarded as the mark of a great scholar!

In China, its use is largely restricted to the Chinese Muslim community, and in such places as Hunan and Xinjiang.

The diminutive seeds pack an extraordinarily hefty punch in terms of flavour and health benefits. With a flavour that resembles caraway seeds, the spice is most commonly used in curry blends for its sweet flavour and in many European foods such as Portuguese sausages, Dutch Leyden cheese and German *sauerkraut*. Cumin is a good source of iron, which is required by the body for producing haemoglobin in the blood, for the proper functioning of enzymes and for manufacturing proteins. Since the ancient times, cumin seeds have been known to promote a healthy digestive system; recent research also suggests that cumin contains anti-oxidants to protect against cancer.

Basic Curry Paste

Integral to the holy trinity with coriander and fenugreek, cumin adds the requisite bitter-sweet spice to curry powder.

Preparation time: 10 minutes
Serves 4

Ground coriander 2 Tbsp
Ground fenugreek 1 Tbsp
Ground cumin 2 tsp
Ground turmeric 1 tsp
Chilli powder 1 tsp
Ginger purée 1 Tbsp
Garlic purée 1 Tbsp
Water 3 Tbsp
Cooking oil 120 ml (4 fl oz / ¹/₂ cup)

Separately dry-fry all ground spices and chilli powder over low heat for about 5 minutes each.

Combine all dry-fried ingredients in a mixing bowl and blend (process) with ginger, garlic and water into a paste.

Heat oil in a wok or pan and fry paste over medium heat until oil separates. Cool and store in a jar. This amount is sufficient for about 3 kg (6 lb 9 oz) of meat or poultry.

Chicken Curry

This is the most basic of Singapore curries and requires very little effort once you have prepared the curry paste.

Preparation time: 20 minutes
Cooking time: 45 minutes
Serves 4–6

Coconut milk 800 ml
(26 fl oz / 3¹/₄ cups) or to taste

Chicken 1.5 kg (3 lb 4¹/₂ oz), cleaned, trimmed of excess fat and cut into large joints

Potatoes 600 g (1 lb 5 oz), peeled and quartered

Basic curry paste 3 Tbsp

Salt 2 tsp

Sugar 2 tsp

Kaffir lime leaves (optional) 6

Pour coconut milk into a pot; use more or less depending on how liquid or thick you like your curry. Add all remaining ingredients and kaffir lime leaves, if using.

Bring to the boil and simmer, covered, over medium heat for about 45 minutes. Check occasionally and stir through to make sure there is no scorching; coconut milk burns easily if you do not use a heavy-bottomed or non-stick pot. Serve hot with rice or bread.

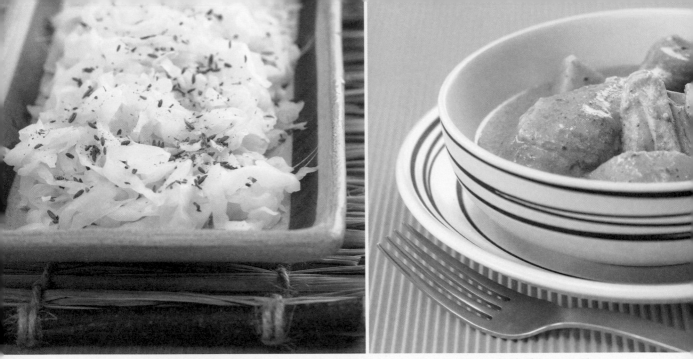

FROM LEFT TO RIGHT: Pickled Cabbage (page 74), Chicken Curry (page 73), Treatment: Tea for Flatulence (page 74)

Pickled Cabbage

Pickled cabbage or *sauerkraut* is the lifeblood of German meals. Its German name literally means 'bitter herb'; the dish originated from the Alsace region, but became synonymous with cooking of the Black Forest and Bavaria in Germany. Traditionally, *sauerkraut* is fermented for a few weeks in a mixture of salt and juniper berries. This version is modified and ready to eat in a day.

Preparation time: 20 minutes
Fermentation time: 2 hours
Cooking time: 10 minutes
Serves 4–6

White cabbage 1 kg (2 lb 3 oz)
Salt 2 Tbsp
White vinegar 2 litres (64 fl oz / 8 cups)
Cumin seeds 1 Tbsp

Shred cabbage but do not wash. Wipe dry with paper towels. Place in a large, dry earthenware or ceramic pot and sprinkle salt all over. Toss well and cover to sweat for 2 hours.

After the sweating period, drain cabbage in colander and squeeze handfuls to remove as much moisture as possible.

Bring vinegar to the boil and blanch cabbage. Drain and place in a serving bowl.

Dry-fry cumin seeds until fragrant and crush lightly. Sprinkle over cabbage. Serve with boiled meats, sausages or roast chicken.

Treatments
Chewing a handful of cumin seeds not only helps to relieve indigestion, but also refresh the mouth after a meal of rich, spicy food. To brew **a tea for treating excesssive flatulence**, crush 1 tsp cumin seeds and infuse with 250 ml (8 fl oz / 1 cup) boiling water for a spicy, carminative drink.

Aromatherapy
Cumin oil is warm and spicy and helps remove stale odours in a room.

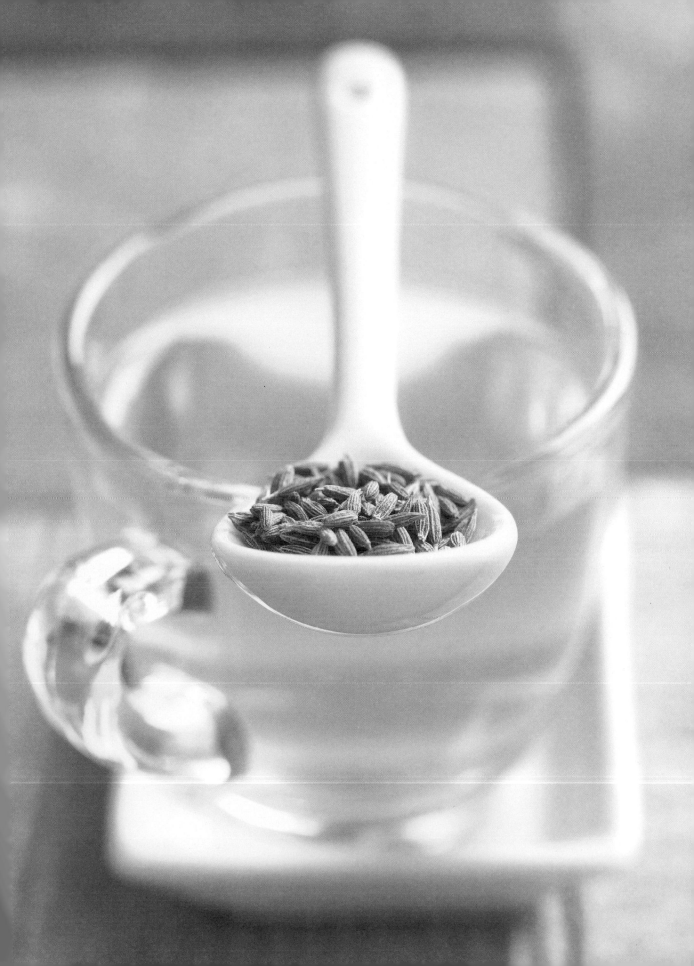

Common Fennel
Mandarin Hui xiang
Cantonese Wui heong
Botanical Foeniculum vulgare

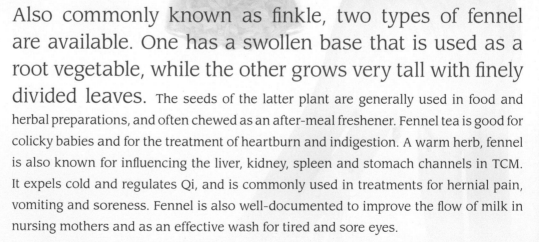

Also commonly known as finkle, two types of fennel are available. One has a swollen base that is used as a root vegetable, while the other grows very tall with finely divided leaves. The seeds of the latter plant are generally used in food and herbal preparations, and often chewed as an after-meal freshener. Fennel tea is good for colicky babies and for the treatment of heartburn and indigestion. A warm herb, fennel is also known for influencing the liver, kidney, spleen and stomach channels in TCM. It expels cold and regulates Qi, and is commonly used in treatments for hernial pain, vomiting and soreness. Fennel is also well-documented to improve the flow of milk in nursing mothers and as an effective wash for tired and sore eyes.

Hippocrates recommended fennel oil for its anti-spasmodic and anti-bacterial qualities. Sweet fennel oil has a very earthy, anise-like aroma due to its primary constituent, anethol. It has a balancing effect on the female reproductive system and increases the flow of body energy.

Fennel, Coriander and Celery Soup

This is a 'green' soup, in that it uses only the bulb, stem and leaves of the fennel. Celery is an effective herb for relieving arthritis. It also acts as a mild diuretic that relieves water retention in PMS.

Preparation time: 10 minutes
Cooking time: 20 minutes
Serves 4

Cooking oil 2 Tbsp

Garlic 2 cloves, crushed

Water 1 litre (32 fl oz / 4 cups)

Vegetable stock cube 1

Fennel bulb 1, whole, sliced

**Coriander leaves
   (cilantro)** 30 g (1 oz), chopped

Celery 2 stalks, thinly sliced

Garnishing

**Chopped celery or
   coriander leaves (cilantro)**

Heat oil in a pan and fry garlic until light brown. Transfer to a pot and add water, stock cube, fennel, coriander and celery.

Simmer for 20 minutes and serve hot, garnished with chopped celery or coriander leaves.

Fennel, Coriander and Celery Soup (page 77)

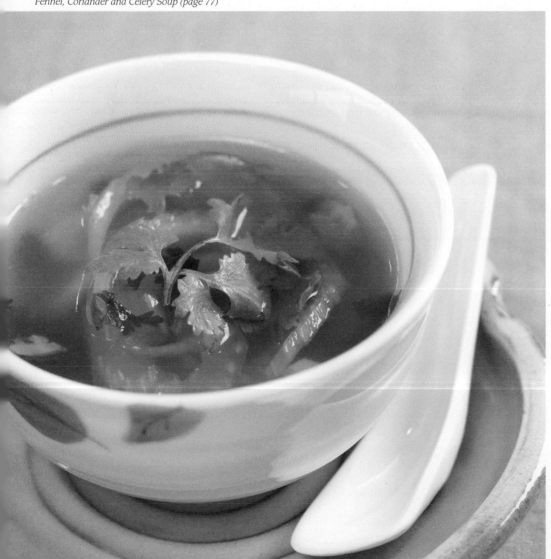

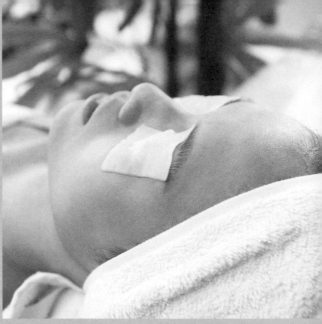

Beauty: Soothing Eye Mask (page 78)

Fennel Rice Wine with Apricot Kernels

This is a warming tonic that helps to relieve hernial pain, promote circulation as well as strengthen kidney and bladder functions.

Preparation time: 25 minutes
Serves 4

Spring onions (scallions) 20 g (²/₃ oz), use white portions only

Bitter apricot kernels 20 g (²/₃ oz), rinsed and thoroughly dried

Sweet apricot kernels 20 g (²/₃ oz), rinsed and thoroughly dried

Fennel seeds 40 g (1¹/₃ oz), rinsed and thoroughly dried

Chinese rice wine

Dry-roast spring onions over low heat until all moisture is removed, until they look browned and shrivelled.

Grind all ingredients except rice wine together into a moist powder.

To drink, stir and dissolve 1 Tbsp powder in 180 ml (6 fl oz / ³/₄ cup) rice wine. Take this portion twice a day.

Treatments

For a herbal infusion, pour 250 ml (8 fl oz / 1 cup) boiling hot water over 1 tsp bruised fennel seeds. Leave to steep for 10 minutes before drinking. It is good for earaches, toothaches, coughs and asthma.

Aromatherapy

Fennel essential oil has been known to aid patients in post-chemotherapy and people with sluggish metabolism. Blend it with a base oil like apricot or almond and use as a massage oil or in a burner. Blend a few drops of fennel oil with almond or lavender oil to use as a massage oil. It helps the flow of body energy and brings the female reproductive system back into balance.

Beauty

Pour 150 ml (5 fl oz / ⁵/₈ cup) boiling hot water onto 3 Tbsp fresh fennel leaves or crushed fennel seeds, and leave to steep for 10 minutes to make an infusion. To soothe irritated skin, dip pieces of cotton wads in fennel infusion and leave on skin until cold. For a **soothing eye mask**, simply place cotton wads dipped in infusion on tired eyes for 15 minutes. To make a relaxing **fennel facial mask**, strain infusion and mix with 100 g (3¹/₂ oz) plain yoghurt. Spread mixture on face and leave on for 15 minutes, then rinse off with warm water.

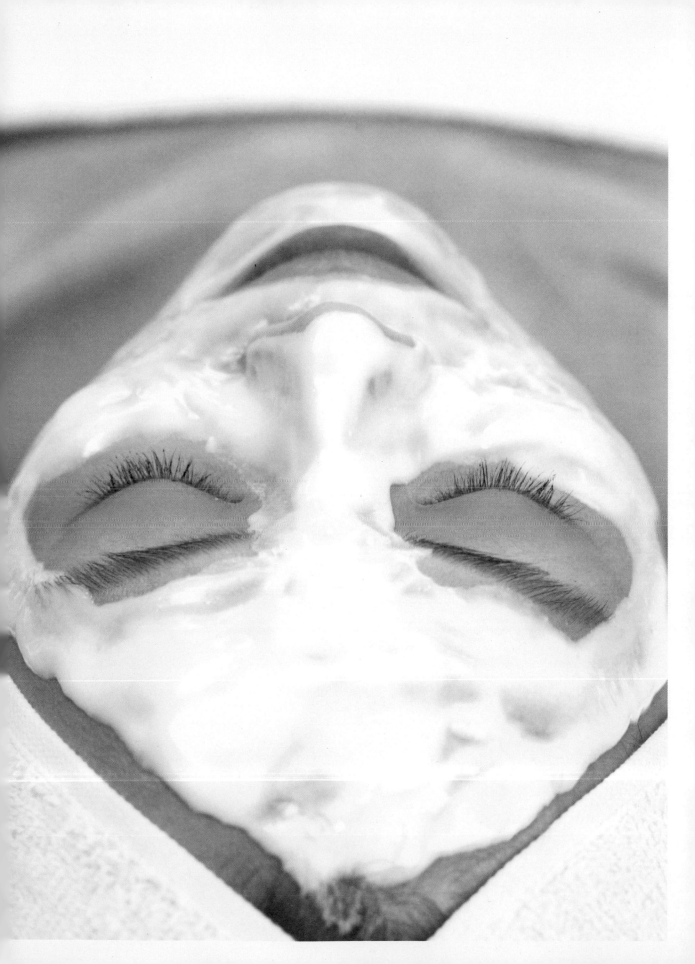

Fenugreek

Common Fenugreek
Mandarin Hu lu ba cai
Cantonese Wu loh ba choyr
Botanical Trigonella foenum-graecum

The name of the spice means 'Greek hay' and the seeds have been used since the ancient times as an aromatic cooking ingredient and medicine by the Greeks, Egyptians, Romans and Chinese. Fenugreek is also a useful source of vitamins and minerals, particularly calcium. The leaves are used more as a culinary ingredient, but have also been documented as an aid for digestion and dispelling wind. Believed to be good for the treatment of kidney ailments, dampness, beriberi and impotence, fenugreek seeds contain volatile oils, mucilage and alkaloids that are known to have carminative, expectorant and laxative actions.

The plant also has therapeutic possibilities that are attributed to its content of steroidal saponins which resemble the body's sex hormones. The steroid-like action of the saponins are believed to be beneficial for menopausal problems and breast enhancement.

Honey Lemon Tea with Crushed Fenugreek Seeds (page 82)

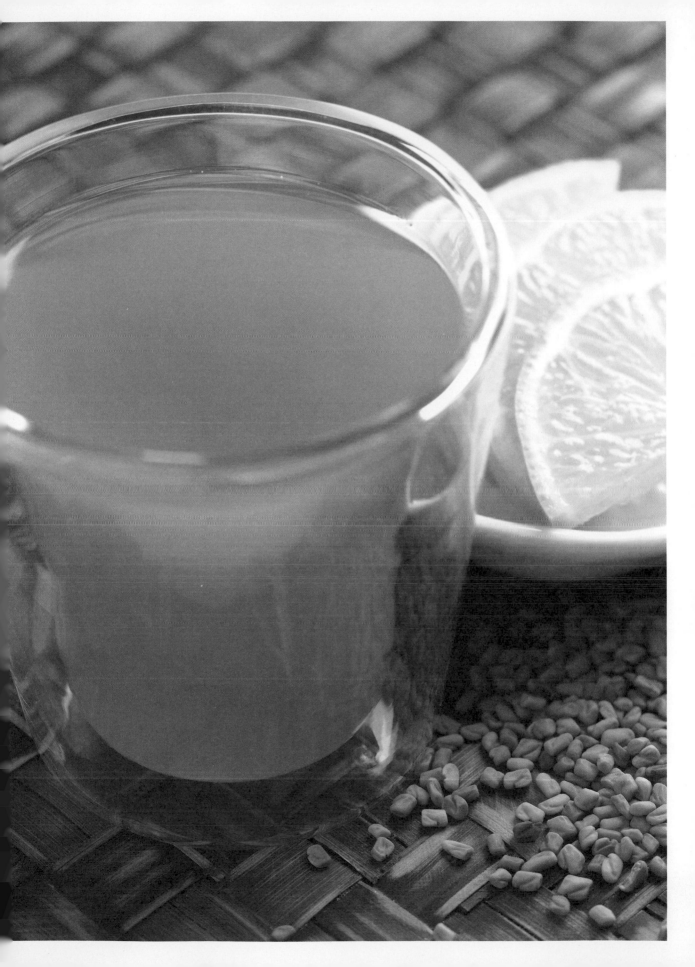

Fenugreek and Mint Tisane

Either the seeds or the very fresh, young shoots of fenugreek can be used to prepare this beverage. Using the leaves, however, can make the drink taste quite bitter, so add a little honey to counter it. Generally, when making a tisane, the ratio is 1 tsp dried herbs to 500 ml (16 fl oz / 2 cups) water. This tisane helps women with low oestrogen levels, especially during menopause.

Preparation time: 10 minutes
Cooking time: 25 minutes
Serves 4

Water 750 ml (24 fl oz / 3 cups)

Fenugreek seeds 40 g (1¼ oz)

Fresh mint leaves 30 g (1 oz)
+ extra for garnishing

Combine all ingredients in a pot and bring to the boil. Remove from heat and leave to steep for 25 minutes.

Strain and discard solid ingredients. Serve warm, garnished with fresh mint leaves.

Fish Curry with Fenugreek Leaves

Fenugreek leaves are a popular green among Indian cooks, to whom they are known as *methi*.

Preparation time: 10 minutes
Cooking time: 20 minutes
Serves 4

Tamarind pulp 2 Tbsp

Warm water 150 ml (5 fl oz / ⅝ cup)

Cooking oil 2 Tbsp

Cumin seeds 1 tsp

Onion 1, large, peeled and chopped

Water 250 ml (8 fl oz / 1 cup)

Threadfin (*ikan kurau*) 500 g
(1 lb 1½ oz), cut into large chunks

Fenugreek leaves 100 g (3½ oz),
stems discarded, washed and drained

Salt 1 tsp

Sugar 1 tsp

Spice Paste

Garlic 2 cloves, peeled

Ginger 3 slices

Chopped coriander 2 Tbsp

Red chillies 2

Knead tamarind pulp with warm water until dissolved. Strain and set aside.

Combine all spice paste ingredients in a blender (processor) and blend (process) until smooth. Set aside.

Heat oil in a wok over medium-high heat. Add cumin seeds and onion and fry for 3 minutes, stirring constantly, until onion is light brown.

Add spice paste and fry until fragrant. Pour in water and bring to the boil, then add half the tamarind liquid, fish, fenugreek leaves, salt and sugar. Cover and simmer for 6–8 minutes. Adjust to taste with more salt or tamarind liquid, if desired. When ready, curry gravy should be thick, full-flavoured and lightly tangy. Serve hot with rice.

Note: This curry can be made with any firm-fleshed white fish. If you cannot find fresh fenugreek leaves, look for packs of frozen chopped leaves in Indian supermarkets and grocery stores. These will work equally well, and save you the trouble of de-stemming them. Simply thaw and squeeze out any excess liquid, then weigh and use.

Treatments

Crush 60 g (2 oz) fenugreek seeds and mix with 2 Tbsp water, then use as poultice on skin irritations, boils and abscesses. **Honey lemon tea with crushed fenugreek seeds** is helpful for digestive problems. Simply infuse 1 tsp crushed fenugreek seeds in 250 ml (8 fl oz / 1 cup) hot lemon tea, then strain and drink.

Beauty

For a **rejuvenating hair and body mask**, simply crush 1 Tbsp fenugreek seeds and mix with (3⅓ fl oz / ⅜ cup) almond oil for a mixture that acts as a stimulant to improve skin and hair. Apply onto damp hair or body. Rinse off after 15 minutes, and shampoo or shower as per usual. Fenugreek has a stimulating effect on the uterus and should not be used during pregnancy.

Rejuvenating Hair and Body Mask (page 82)

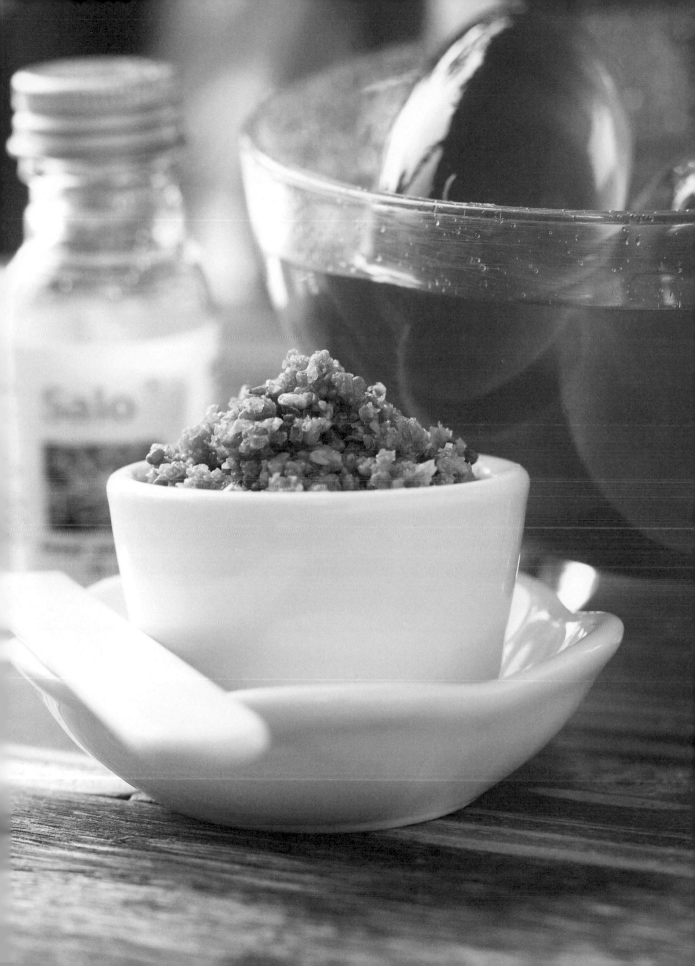

Foxglove Root

The plant is grown in north and northwest China, and it is the tuberous root or rhizome that is used. The pieces of the root are rather nondescript in appearance: black and hardened clumps. In its fresh and untreated form, the root is called *sheng di huang* in Mandarin or *sang tei wong* in Cantonese, both of which translate into 'raw earth'. The treated form is known respectively as *shou di huang* in Mandarin, or *sok tei wong* in Cantonese, meaning 'cooked earth'. To 'cook' the 'earth', pieces of the root are dried in a kiln. Foxglove root is believed to be good for the treatment of coughs, headaches, vertigo, low blood pressure, backache, threatened miscarriage, inflamed eyes and anaemia, as well as disorders of the kidneys and lungs.

Common Foxglove root
Mandarin Di huang
Cantonese Tei wong
Botanical Rehmannia glutinosa

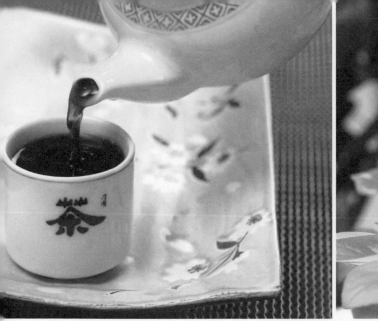
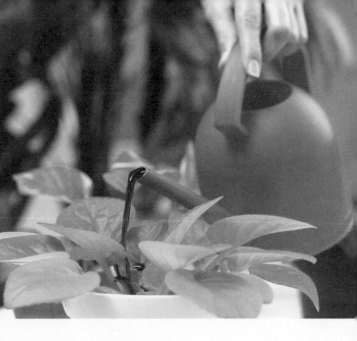

FROM LEFT TO RIGHT: Youthful Tea (page 85), Natural Insect Spray (page 85)

Youthful Tea

The combination of foxglove and Chinese angelica is reputedly good for young girls' development. It helps to nourish the blood, relieve menstrual cramps and check irregular menstruation.

Preparation time: 15 minutes
Cooking time: 25 minutes
Serves 4

Water 1 litre (32 fl oz / 4 cups)

Treated foxglove root 10 g (¹/₃ oz), rinsed and drained

Chinese angelica 10 g (¹/₃ oz), rinsed and drained

Combine all ingredients in a pot and simmer for 1 hour, then strain and serve immediately.

Natural Insect Spray

Foxglove root 50 g (2 oz)

Water 400 ml (13 fl oz)

Boil foxglove root in water and cool completely.

Use cooled liquid as a spray to deter pests on household plants. Make a large amount and use it to water outdoor plants to deter ants, greenflies and whiteflies.

Chicken, Angelica and Foxglove Root Soup

Preparation time: 20 minutes
Cooking time: 1 hour
Serves 4

Chicken 1, about 1.5 kg (3 lb 4¹/₂ oz), cleaned and trimmed of excess fat

Treated foxglove root 20 g (²/₃ oz), rinsed and drained

Chinese angelica 20 g (²/₃ oz), rinsed and drained

Water 1 litre (32 fl oz / 4 cups)

Salt 2 tsp

Combine all ingredients in a pot, then cover and simmer for 1 hour.

Remove herbs before serving soup and chicken.

Garlic

Virtually a universal panacea, garlic needs little introduction and has been highly prized for millennia. Its versatility knows few bounds and its curative properties are now legion, except for those with a preternatural dislike for the bulb.

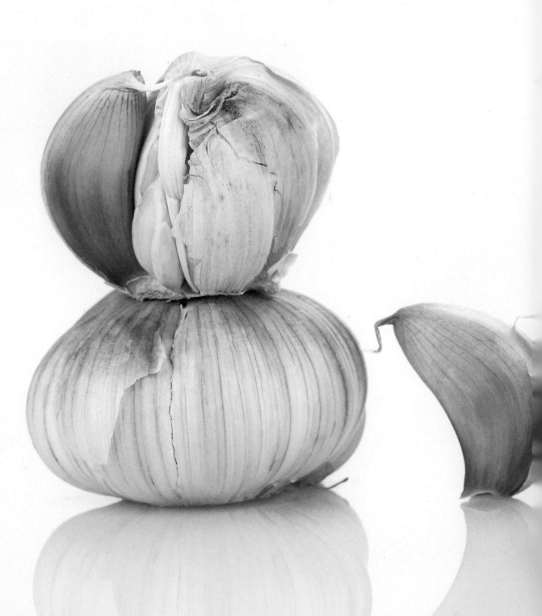

Garlic is as much a curative ingredient as it is a masterly culinary one known for its pungency, vitamins, flavonoids, proteins and oils. A virtual powerhouse, garlic has anti-inflammatory, antibiotic, expectorant and anti-microbial actions, and modern clinical tests have shown that regular use of garlic helps to thin the blood, lower cholesterol levels and alleviate high blood pressure. Its strong odour is due to the presence of sulphur compounds. It also helps to improve circulation, fight off infection and ward off colds, sinusitis and sore throats. The ancient Egyptians knew of its efficacy as far back as 1500 b.c., and during World War I, it was used extensively to reduce wound infections.

To derive maximum benefit from garlic, use it or eat it raw as cooking breaks down many of its active ingredients. Taken orally, garlic capsules may increase the effects of anti-coagulant and blood-thinning medication. Garlic essential oil helps to relieve tiredness and stimulate cell production as well as promote blood circulation.

Chicken with Garlic in Black Bean Sauce

Preparation time: 15 minutes
Cooking time: 10 minutes
Serves 4

Vegetable oil 2 Tbsp

Garlic 4 cloves, peeled and crushed

Chicken breast 350 g (12 oz), thinly sliced

Black bean sauce 2 Tbsp

Chinese cooking wine (*shao hsing*) 3 Tbsp

Sugar 2 tsp

Sesame oil 2 Tbsp

Ground white pepper to taste

Water 100 ml (3$\frac{1}{3}$ fl oz / $\frac{3}{8}$ cup)

Heat oil and fry sliced garlic until light brown. Push aside and add chicken to the pan to stir-fry over high heat for 2 minutes.

Add black bean sauce, Chinese cooking wine, sugar, sesame oil, pepper to taste and water. Stir over high heat for 1–2 minutes, or until sauce is thick. Dish out and serve hot.

Garlic and Bean Curd Soup

This soup is not for the faint-hearted but will be loved by garlic fans. You may even double the amount of garlic for healthy measure. It is a full-bodied and aromatic soup, ideal for vegetarians.

Preparation time: 10 minutes
Cooking time: 15 minutes
Serves 4

Light chicken or vegetable stock 1 litre (32 fl oz / 4 cups)

Garlic 10 cloves, peeled and thinly sliced

Cloves 6

Silken bean curd 250 g (9 oz), cut into small dice

Vegetable stock cube 1

Chopped spring onions (scallions) 2 Tbsp

Ground black pepper 1 tsp

Bring stock to the boil in a pot. Add garlic cloves and simmer for 5–6 minutes.

Remove garlic slices with a slotted spoon and discard — you may leave some in the soup to eat or for garnish, if desired. Add bean curd, reduce heat to low and simmer very gently for 10 minutes more.

Serve hot, garnished with spring onions and pepper.

Note: Add 100 g (3¹/₃ oz) of very thinly sliced chicken or pork if a more substantial soup is desired.

Treatments

There are many garlic pills and capsules available in the market, that can be taken orally to help increase the effects of anti-coagulant and blood-thinning medication. **Garlic capsules** are also said to be good for lowering the cholesterol level and amount of fats in the body as well as strengthening the immune system. To reduce the risk of infection for wounds, apply **a poultice of raw ground garlic** on the affected area for several hours.

Aromatherapy

Garlic essential oil has stimulating qualities. It not only relieves tiredness, but also helps to stimulate blood circulation and cell production within the lymphatic system. Mix with a fragrant base oil, such as sweet almond, to neutralise the strong odour of garlic.

CLOCKWISE FROM TOP: Garlic and Bean Curd Soup (page 88), Treatments: Raw Garlic Poultice (page 88), Garlic Capsules (page 88)

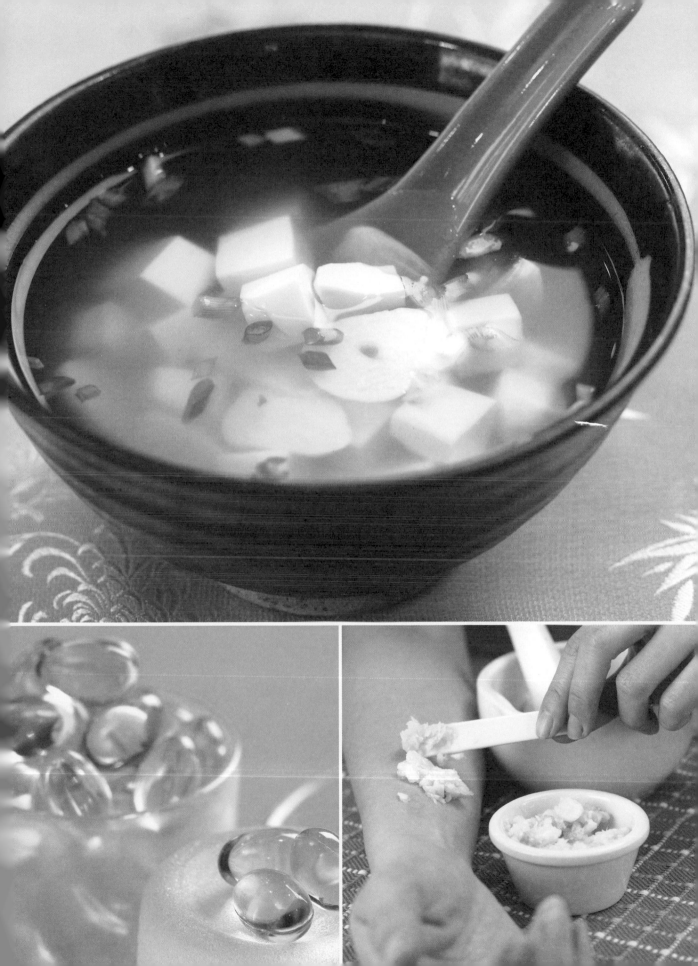

Ginger

A herbaceous perennial plant consisting of an underground stem or rhizome from which leafy shoots grow to about one metre in height, ginger is probably the oldest spice known in the east. It was only taken to America and Europe in the 16th century and remains a favourite kitchen herb.

As a medicinal ingredient, ginger has been known for its medicinal properties for thousands of years and for its warm action across a wide range of treatments. Only the dried or fresh root is used for its volatile oil and resin, and for its aromatic, carminative and expectorant actions. Ginger helps to improve digestion, reduce flatulence and colic. It is also known for its efficacy in alleviating motion sickness and bronchial problems. In aromatherapy, ginger essential oil is used as a massage oil for relieving pain and healing bone injuries.

Common Ginger
Mandarin Jiang
Cantonese Keong
Botanical Zingiber officinale

Egg Drop and Ginger Soup with Prawns

This classic Cantonese soup is warming and delicious, either as a late snack or a starter soup.

Preparation time: 10 minutes
Cooking time: 10 minutes
Serves 4

Water 800 ml (26 fl oz / 3¹/₄ cups)

Ginger 30 g (1 oz), peeled and finely julienned

Crushed garlic 1 Tbsp

Ground black pepper 1 tsp

Chinese cooking wine (*shao hsing*) 3 Tbsp

Salt 2 tsp

Prawns 150 g (5 oz), shelled and deveined

Eggs 2, lightly beaten

Coriander leaves (cilantro) 20 g (²/₃ oz)

Bring water to the boil in a pot. Add ginger and garlic and simmer for 5 minutes.

Add pepper, wine, salt and prawns. Simmer for 3 minutes, then slowly pour in beaten egg in one continuous stream while stirring.

Cook for 1 minute more and serve, garnished with coriander.

Spare Ribs with Ginger and Garlic

To get the best results for spare ribs, I recommend that you boil them in their marinade before grilling them briefly. This ensures that the ribs effectively absorb the marinade and are moist and succulent.

Preparation time: 30 minutes
Cooking time: 45 minutes
Serves 4

Pork spare ribs 500 g (1 lb 1¹/₂ oz), cleaned, trimmed of excess fat and cut into large pieces

Marinade

Ginger purée 2 Tbsp

Garlic purée 2 Tbsp

Hoi sin sauce 2 Tbsp

Preserved red bean curd (*nam yee*) 1 cube

Chinese cooking wine (*shao hsing*) 100 ml (3¹/₂ fl oz)

Sugar 1 Tbsp

Water 700 ml (23 fl oz / 2³/₄ cups)

Salt 2 tsp

Combine all marinade ingredients in a pot and stir until well-blended. Mix in ribs and leave to marinate for about 1 hour.

Bring ribs and marinade to the boil and cook over high heat for 45 minutes; this will take 30 minutes in a pressure cooker.

Transfer ribs to a roasting pan and oven-grill them for 10 minutes or until they char a little. Serve hot.

Note: Any excess marinade can be used a second time if you chill or freeze it.

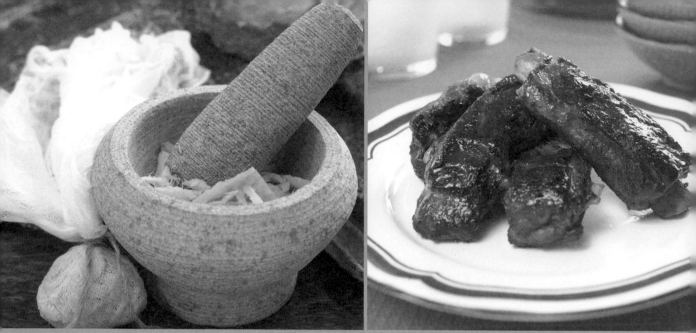

FROM LEFT TO RIGHT: Poultice for Rheumatic Pain (page 92), Spare Ribs with Ginger and Garlic (page 91), Ginger Slices for Indigestion (page 92)

Ginger and Cardamom Tea

This is the simplest brew that helps to dispel dyspepsia and boost sluggish appetites.

Preparation time: 30 minutes
Cooking time: 45 minutes
Serves 4

Ginger 30 g (1 oz), peeled
Cardamom 6 pods
Water 800 ml (26 fl oz / 3¹/₄ cups)
Rock sugar 30 g (1 oz)

Combine all ingredients in a pot and bring to the boil, then simmer for 15 minutes.

Strain to remove solid ingredients and drink it hot.

Treatments

As a child I remember being treated with a poultice of crushed and heated ginger for all manner of ills, mainly to do with the stomach. It is especially good for inducing perspiration and dispersing cold. Crush a large knob of ginger and boil in 1 litre water for 10 minutes. Allow to cool until it can be tolerated by the body and wash all over to induce perspiration for the relief of fever.

To make a **poultice for rheumatic pain**, wrap 2 Tbsp crushed ginger in a clean piece of muslin or cotton gauze and warm in a microwave oven on high for 1 minute. Apply on affected area for relief, for about an hour.

For indigestion, simply chew on a **thin, peeled slice of fresh ginger** before swallowing. Take this remedy 2 to 3 times a day until symptoms subside.

Ginger root is also widely available in capsule form, and can be taken for treating the ailments mentioned earlier, including rheumatism and indigestion. Most capsules contain four percent volatile oil. Instant packets of ginger tea are also readily available at Chinese medicinal shops for relieving colds, nausea and gastric discomfort.

Aromatherapy

Ginger essential oil can be used as part of a massage oil blend for pain and bone injuries, when blended with a base oil like sweet almond or apricot. It is also highly recommended for muscle fatigue and sports injuries. For the relief of conditions including backaches, rheumatism and painful joints, various Chinese brands of ginger massage oil are also available for treatment.

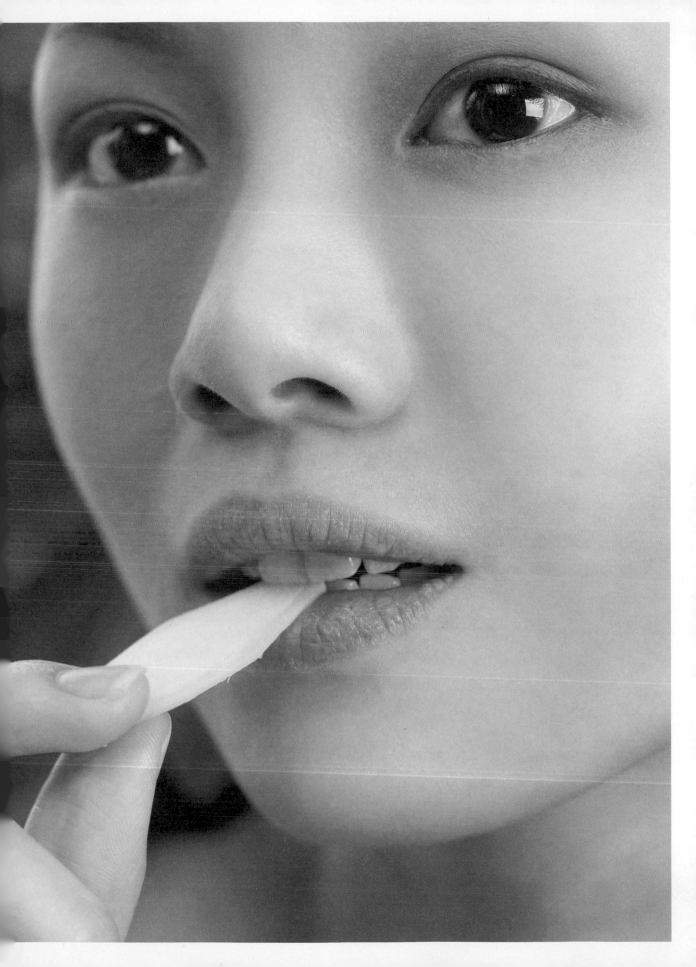

Gingko Nut

Common Gingko nut
Mandarin Bai guo
Cantonese Bahk gor
Botanical Gingko bilobae semen

Also known as the maidenhair tree, the gingko plant dates back some 2 million years and is revered as a tree of life in Asia for its remarkable properties. Native to Japan and the Chinese provinces of Guangxi, Sichuan and Henan, the nuts are good for asthma, coughs, gynaecological problems, bladder ailments and urinary disorders. An extract of the fruit is supposed to have a strongly deterrent effect on the growth of bacteria-causing tuberculosis. Gingko nuts are also known to have anti-oxidant and anti-allergic qualities, improve circulation and enhance energy metabolism in the brain.

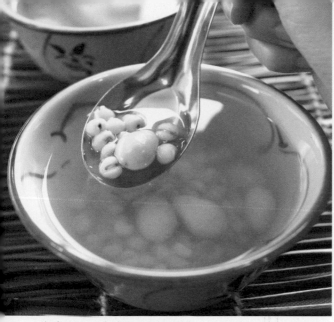
Gingko Nuts and Job's Tears (page 95)

Gingko Nuts and Job's Tears

In TCM, gingko nuts are believed to strengthen the bladder and address related ailments. This 'cooling' brew is also known to offset the detrimental effects of having eaten too many 'hot' foods.

Preparation time: 15 minutes
Cooking time: 1 hour
Serves 4

Job's tears 3 Tbsp, washed and drained

Screwpine (pandan) leaves 2

Water 2 litres (64 fl oz / 8 cups)

Precooked gingko nuts 40–50,

Rock sugar 140 g (4 1/2 oz)

Combine Job's tears, screwpine leaves and water in a pot. Bring to the boil and simmer over medium heat for 40 minutes.

Add gingko nuts and rock sugar. Simmer for 20 minutes more, or until gingko nuts are just soft and cooked. Serve warm as a dessert.

Chicken Soup with Winter Melon and Gingko Nuts

This is a traditional northern Chinese dish cooked often during the biting winter months. The tradition of serving hearty herbal soups has remained unchanged for centuries, and is today a dish that still goes down well for its delicious flavour.

Preparation time: 20 minutes
Cooking time: 45 minutes
Serves 4

Chicken 1.5 kg (3 lb 4 1/2 oz), cleaned and cut into 8 joints

Water 2 litres (64 fl oz / 8 cups)

Winter melon 450 g (1 lb), peeled, pith removed and cut into chunks

Precooked gingko nuts 40

Salt 2 tsp

Combine chicken and water in a pot. Bring to a simmer and cook slowly for 40 minutes.

Add winter melon and gingko nuts, and simmer for another 20 minutes, then add salt.

To save time, pressure-cook chicken in water for 30 minutes, then add winter melon and gingko nuts. Continue to pressure-cook for 15 minutes. Serve hot.

Note: If using dried gingko nuts, they should be soaked for several hours and added for the entire pressure-cooking time.

Ginseng

Common Ginseng
Mandarin Ren shen
Cantonese Yam sam
Botanical Panax ginseng

This strange-looking root has been regarded by the Chinese and other Asians for hundreds of years as the universal panacea. No other natural product quite matches it for the reputation of being a super restorative.

Today, ginseng is widely accepted as belonging to one of three main types — Chinese ginseng (*ren shen / yan sam*); American ginseng (*yang shen/yong sam*); and Korean ginseng (*gao li shen / go lai sam*). American ginseng is sometimes also known as 'flower-flag' ginseng (*hua qi shen / fa kei sam*) because the Chinese in the past likened the numerous stars on the American flag to flowers.

Within each type of ginseng, however, are many grades, and it is the grade that matters more. Also, the name of the root no longer indicates the geographical origins of the root, but only its species. The lucrative and curative promise of the revered root has spurred growers around the world to try their hand at cultivating any faintly profitable species of ginseng. China, to that end, is the world's largest exporter of American ginseng. Far less important than where the root comes from is how it came to be; wild ginseng is always infinitely more valuable than its farmed counterpart.

Much research has been done on this most famous of Chinese herbs in an effort to discover the secrets that reside within. Since the mid-twentieth century, the root has been examined thoroughly, and several physiologically active substances have been isolated — in particular *panaxin* which increases muscular tone; *panax acid* which improves metabolism and the vascular system; *panaquilon* which influences the endocrine system; *panacen* which stimulates the nerve centres; and *ginsenin* which is supposed to be beneficial for diabetes sufferers — thereby lending some strength to the once disputed beliefs that ginseng invigorates and also encourages healing processes in the body after illness.

The vast number of properties in ginseng gives an almost unlimited use in cosmetics. Nourishing creams help in the treatment of wrinkles and retardation of ageism. In body milks and bath products, ginseng acts by optimizing the cutaneous metabolism of the whole body, and in capillary products, ginseng is used in the treatment of weak hair and hair loss.

Chicken and Ginseng

Obviously the type of ginseng you use is entirely of personal taste and pocket.

Preparation time: 20 minutes
Cooking time: 1 hour
Serves 4

Chicken 1, about 1.5 kg (3 lb 4 1/2 oz), cleaned and trimmed of excess fat

Ginseng 20 g (3/4 oz), rinsed and drained

Water 1 litre (32 fl oz / 4 cups)

Salt 2 tsp

Combine all ingredients in a pot and simmer, covered, for 1 hour. Serve hot.

Note: The chicken meat will have been rendered relatively bland, but still retains some nutrition. It is best deboned and eaten with a sharp or salty sauce.

Ginseng and Bird's Nest

Whatever grade ginseng you choose, remember that it is a potent herb and a little goes a long way. Dr. Geng recommends that ginseng should not be taken by those with high blood pressure. Otherwise, herbalists swear by ginseng for good health, glowing hair and a sparkling disposition.

Preparation time: 20 minutes
Cooking time: 1 hour
Serves 4

Ginseng 15 g (1/2 oz), rinsed and drained

Bird's nest 50 g (2 oz), thoroughly cleaned

Rock sugar 140 g (5 oz)

Water 1.5 litres (48 fl oz / 6 cups)

Rinse ginseng and drain. Combine all ingredients in a pot and simmer for about 1 hour. Serve hot or cold as a dessert.

Chicken with Dates and Korean Ginseng

Korean ginseng is known as *gao li shen* in Mandarin, and *goh lai sum* in Cantonese. It is quite similar to Chinese ginseng — r*en shen* (Mandarin); *yan sum* (Cantonese) — but is regarded as having more potency.

Preparation time: 20 minutes
Cooking time: 1 hour
Serves 4

Chicken 1, about 900 g (2 lb), cleaned and trimmed of excess fat

Dried Chinese red dates 15, pitted, rinsed and drained

Korean ginseng 60 g (2 oz), rinsed and drained

Water 1 litre (32 fl oz / 4 cups)

Salt 2 tsp or to taste

Combine all ingredients in a pot and simmer for about 1 hour.

Taste soup and adjust seasoning to taste with more salt, if required. When you are satisfied with the taste and consistency of your precious soup, you absolutely must serve it in the finest porcelain.

Treatments

To relieve 'heatiness' and strengthen the immune system, **instant sachets of ginseng tea** are readily available at many Chinese medicinal shops. Some manufacturers of herbal medicine produce **small vials of liquid ginseng extract** which can be drunk to improve the flow of Qi in the body, relieve fatigue, improve sluggish appetite and treat insomnia. **Ginseng capsules** are now widely available; they purportedly help to improve overall physical well-being as well as relieve general fatigue.

CLOCKWISE FROM CENTRE: Treatments: Ginseng Liquid Extract (page 98), Ginseng Capsules (page 98) and Ginseng Tea Bag (page 98)

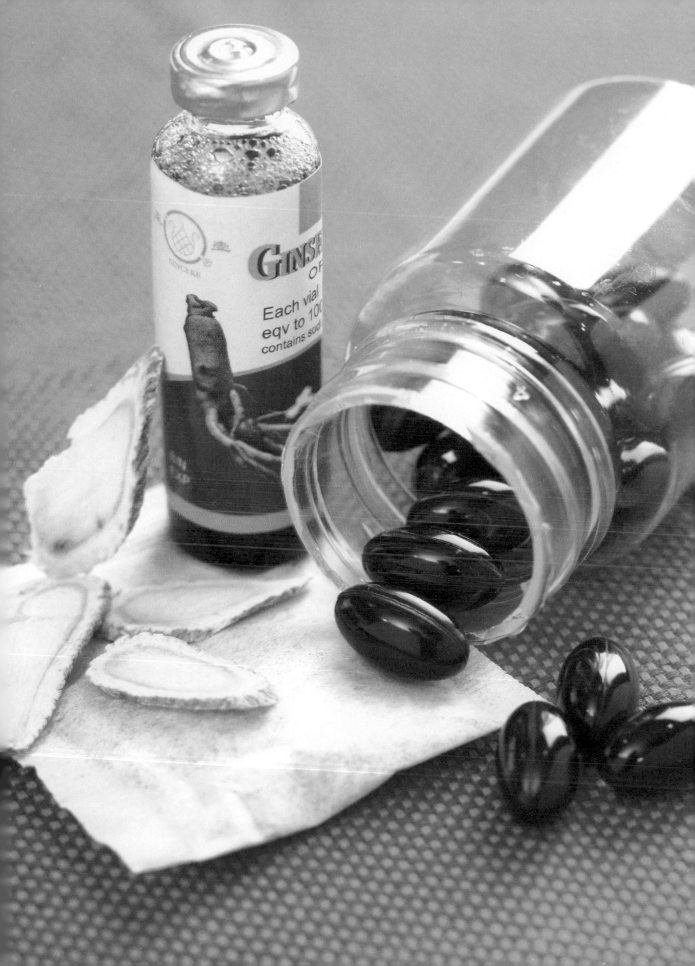

Job's Tear

Common Job's tear, Chinese barley
Mandarin Yi yi ren
Cantonese Yi mai
Botanical Coix lacryma jobi

Job's tear is commonly known as Chinese barley, and has very different properties from the common barley, although it looks and tastes like the latter when cooked. One way to differentiate Job's tears from common barley is that Job's tears do not produce as much mucilaginous substance when boiled in water as common barley.

The kernels of the Chinese barley plant, which grows in India, south China and Papua New Guinea, are separated from their shells and used both as food and medicine throughout Asia. The properties of the Chinese barley are diuretic, spleen-invigorating and heat-dispersing. It helps to ease aching joints, swelling and is a powerful anti-oxidant and tonic. In TCM, it is commonly used in the treatment of rheumatism, edema, warts, eczema, chronic enteritis, diarrhoea, lung abscess, acute appendicitis and even gonorrhea. Reported to inhibit the growth of cancer cells, Job's tears are believed to be especially good for babies and young children when boiled with a little winter melon rind.

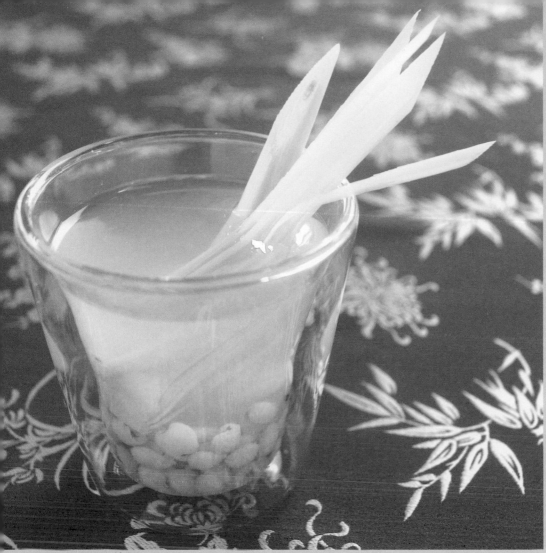

Lemon Grass Tea with Job's Tears (page 101)

Lemon Grass Tea with Job's Tears

This drink is pure inventiveness, courtesy of a Thai friend who swears by it. She also tells me it can treat mild urinary infections as it rids the body of excess heat that causes reduced immunity. At the very least, this drink certainly brings together two mostly unlikely herbal partners, and for mysteriously good Zen synergy.

Preparation time: 10 minutes
Cooking time: 35 minutes
Serves 4

Lemon grass 3 stalks
Job's tears 140 g (5 oz)
Rock sugar 140 g (5 oz)
Water 800 ml (26 fl oz / 3¹/₄ cups)
Vanilla essence (extract) ¹/₂ tsp

Trim leaf end of each lemon grass stalk, leaving about 7.5 cm (3 in) from the bulbous root end. Bruise each stalk lightly with the back of a knife and set aside.

Combine all ingredients in a pot and simmer, covered, over medium heat for about 45 minutes. Regularly skim off froth from the surface. Serve warm.

Treatments
Capsules of ground Job's tears are taken to improve digestion, reduce water retention and also rid the system of excess mucus.

Lemon Grass

Common Lemon grass
Mandarin Feng mao, Ning meng xiang mao
Cantonese Heong maow
Botanical Cymbopogon citratus

This is one herb that transcends cultures, and is probably the best-known kitchen ingredient today that also has efficacious promise. Whether it is used liberally in tom yam soup, or steeped in wine for a unique tipple, lemon grass is useful for improving sluggish digestion.

While not a 'star' within the herbal field, lemon grass is nevertheless blessed with cooling and anti-microbial properties for curing stomach upsets. It is now also available as an aromatherapy oil, useful as a natural deodorizer for the feet and great for use in an aromatherapy burner, to rid a room of cigarette or cigar smoke and other unpleasant smells.

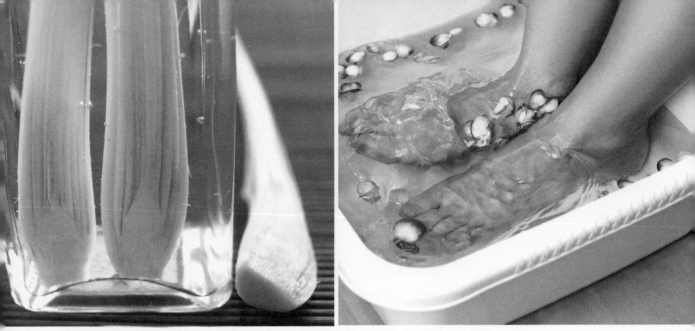

FROM LEFT TO RIGHT: Lemon Grass White Wine (page 103), Treatment: Lemon Grass Relaxing Foot Bath (page 103)

Lemon Grass Prawn Skewers

Apart from its microbial properties, lemon grass is the true chameleon of the herb citrus family. Ground in a spice paste, sliced for stir-frying, or simply used as a fragrant skewer for meat or prawns, it is ambrosial.

Preparation time: 30 minutes
Cooking time: 30 minutes
Serves 4

Lemongrass 16 stalks

Prawns 600 g (1 lb 5 oz), shelled and deveined

Salt 1 tsp

Sugar 1 tsp

Turmeric powder 1 tsp

Coriander powder 1 tbsp

Cumin powder 2 tsp

Cooking oil 1 Tbsp + more for brushing

Egg yolk 1

Trim off leafy end of each lemon grass stalk, leaving about 15–20 cm (6–8 in) in length. Set aside.

Combine prawns, salt, sugar, all ground spices, 1 Tbsp oil and egg yolk in a blender (processor). Pulse until a coarse paste is formed. Do not overwork mixture. Scrape into a bowl, cover, and chill in the coldest part of fridge for 30 minutes.

Divide prawn mixture into 16 equal portions and wrap each one around the base of a lemon grass stalk, patting it firmly to help it adhere.

Grill (broil) prawn sticks over charcoal for about 5 minutes until browned, turning and brushing with more oil frequently. Serve as an amusing starter.

Treatments

After a hard day's foot slogging, soaking your feet in a hot herbal bath can be very rejuvenating. Boil enough water to fill a **foot bath**. Add 2–3 drops of lemon grass essential oil and allow water to cool enough to soak your feet in. It soothes and deodorizes at the same time.

Aromatherapy

Add a few drops of lemon grass oil to a base oil like almond, and use on a burner to perfume a room with its citrus tang. Add a few drops of lemon grass oil to a hot bath and luxuriate in it. Light a few lemon-scented candles and you will float out of there after 20 minutes.

Lemon Grass White Wine

I had occasion to try this in a Thai friend's restaurant in upstate New York some years ago. She simply steeped several stalks of lemon grass in a dry white wine for 2 weeks. The taste is very subtle but definitely lemon grassy and goes very well with Thai dishes.

Preparation time: 5 minutes
Serves 6–8

Dry white wine 1 bottle, 750 ml (24 fl oz / 3 cups)

Lemon grass 3 stalks

Trim off about 5 cm (2 in) from the green, leafy end of each stalk, then wash and dry thoroughly.

Uncork wine and add lemon grass, then reseal as tightly as possible. Given that any opened bottle of wine needs to be drunk fairly quickly, 2 weeks is as long as you can steep. Serve chilled.

Prawns with Lemon Grass and Holy Basil

This dish epitomises Thai stir-fries and is redolent with a lemony-sherberty aroma that is irresistible.

Preparation time: 10 minutes
Cooking time: 5 minutes
Serves 4

Vegetable oil 2 Tbsp

Garlic 2 cloves, peeled and crushed

Lemon grass 3 stalks, use lower 5 cm (2 in) only, thinly sliced on a diagonal

Red chillies 2, sliced

Tiger prawns (shrimps) 450 g (1 lb), shelled and deveined, then washed and drained

Holy basil leaves 30 g (1 oz), chopped

Kalamansi limes 1–2, halved

Sauce (combined)

Fish sauce 1 Tbsp

Sugar 1 tsp

Water 120 ml (4 fl oz)

Cornflour (cornstarch) 1 tsp

Heat oil in a deep pan or wok. Fry garlic, lemon grass and chillies for about 1 minute, then add prawns and stir-fry over high heat until they turn pink.

Add basil leaves and stir-fry for 1 minute before adding well-blended sauce ingredients. Cook, stirring constantly, until sauce is thick.

Dish out and accompany with cut limes for squeezing juice over, if desired. Serve hot with rice and other dishes.

Lemon Grass Prawn Skewers (page 103)

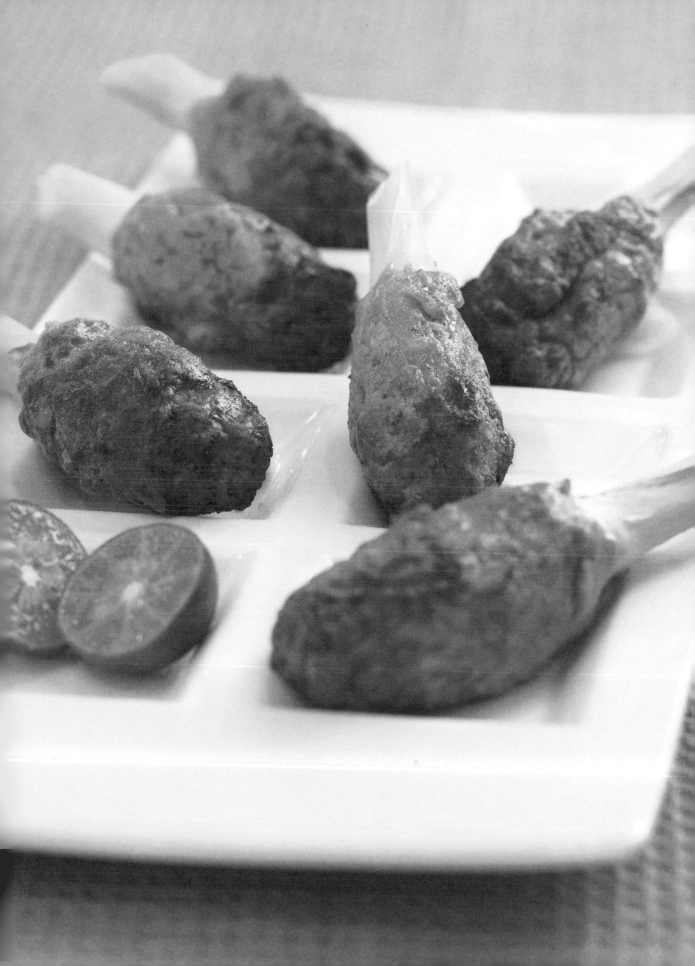

Lily Bulb Petal

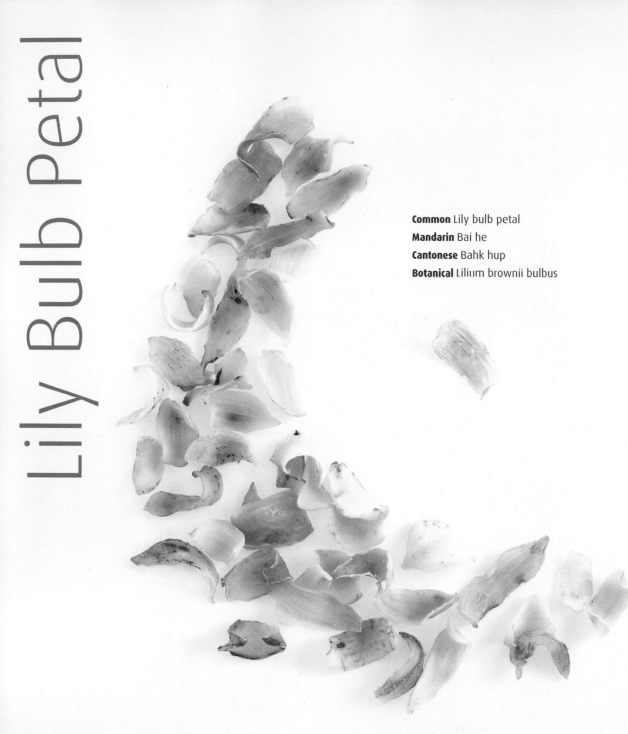

Common Lily bulb petal
Mandarin Bai he
Cantonese Bahk hup
Botanical Lilium brownii bulbus

These are petals of the genus related to the magnolia flower native to China and Vietnam. The bulbs are harvested from July to September, separated, blanched, dried and bleached in sulphur fumes. Lily bulb petals are believed to be beneficial for an extraordinary range of illnesses, from pulmonary diseases and deafness to ulcers and cough. It is a 'cooling' herb that influences the heart and lung channels.

Lily Bulb Petals and Red Date Tea

Red dates are said to prevent skin problems, improve blood circulation and work against cell degeneration. They are also good for masking the less than pleasant flavours of strong-tasting herbs in a given blend. Do not discard the dates after cooking as they are rich in vitamins C and E.

Preparation time: 10 minutes
Cooking time: 40 minutes
Serves 4

Lily bulb petals 55 g (2 oz), washed and drained

Dried Chinese red dates 20, pitted, rinsed and drained

Water 800 ml (26 fl oz / 3¹/₄ cups)

Combine all ingredients in a pot. Bring to the boil and simmer over low heat for 40 minutes. Serve warm or chilled.

Bean Curd with Straw Mushrooms and Lily Bulb Petals

This is a delicious vegetarian option for when you have had a surfeit of meat and other rich dishes. The traditional recipe calls for belly pork but fried squares of firm bean curd make a substantial and healthier choice. The recipe calls for only straw mushrooms, but it does not mean you cannot innovate and use several types, like button and shiitake. Lily bulb petals provide herbal efficacy, and a balance of lightness and fragrance.

Preparation time: 10 minutes
Cooking time: 30 minutes
Serves 4

Firm bean curd (*tau kwa*) 2 pieces

Vegetable oil 2 Tbsp

Canned straw mushrooms 20, drained, rinsed and drained again

Lily bulb petals 15 g (¹/₂ oz), washed and drained

Oyster sauce 2 Tbsp

Hoi sin sauce 1 Tbsp

Salt 1 tsp

Water 400 ml (13 fl oz)

Quarter each piece of bean curd on the diagonal into 4 triangles.

Heat oil in a pan. Add bean curd pieces and fry for 3 minutes or until light brown. Remove and drain on paper towels.

Combine all remaining ingredients including fried bean curd, except water, in a non-stick pot or casserole. Add water until ingredients are completely covered, then simmer over medium heat for 25 minutes. Add small amounts of water, if mixture is dry. Serve hot with rice.

Bean Curd with Straw Mushrooms and Lily Bulb Petals (page 107)

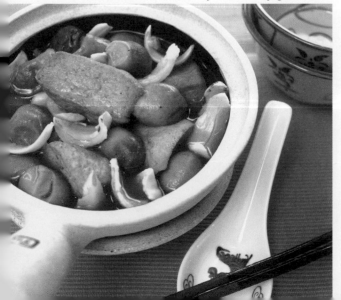

Liquorice

One of the most widely used herbs in Chinese herbal medicine, liquorice has significant anti-viral and anti-bacterial qualities that are useful in combatting common colds and influenza. The root is used for its constituents of glycosides, saponins, bitters, volatile oils and tannins. Its expectorant, anti-arthritic, laxative and demulcent actions help to loosen phlegm, reduce rheumatic inflammation, support Qi, improve sluggish digestion, prevent dryness, clear toxins, relieve heatiness and alleviate pain. The neutral action of the sweet-tasting herb influences the action of

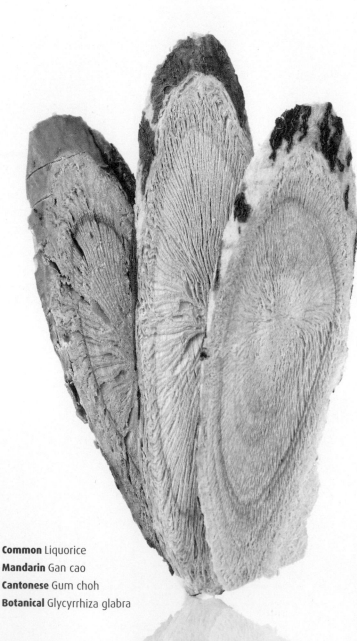

Common Liquorice
Mandarin Gan cao
Cantonese Gum choh
Botanical Glycyrrhiza glabra

the 12 major body channels in Chinese herbalism. It can also be applied topically as a poultice, to relieve cold sores and shingles, and is good for combatting acid build-up in the duodenal area.

Liquorice is included in most Chinese herbal combinations to balance the other herbs and to promote vitality. It has a reputation for bringing the entire body into balance and is particularly beneficial for women with menstruation problems and for promoting general well-being. Today, liquorice is available in capsule form and cream, the latter being effective for the treatment of eczema and psoriasis.

Stir-fried Chicken with Liquorice, Ginger and Turmeric (page 110)

Stir-fried Chicken with Liquorice, Ginger and Turmeric

This a hybrid blend of Thai, Chinese and Malay elements that makes good eating with efficacious promise.

Preparation time: 15 minutes
Cooking time: 15 minutes
Serves 4

Liquorice root slivers 70 g (2¹/₂ oz), finely ground into a powder

Shredded turmeric 1 Tbsp

Vegetable oil 2 Tbsp

Ginger 60 g (2 oz), peeled and julienned

Chicken breast 300 g (11 oz), cut into thin strips

Spring onions (scallions) 2, finely chopped

Light soy sauce 1 Tbsp

Ground black pepper ¹/₂ tsp

Water 180 ml (6 fl oz / ³/₄ cup)

Mix liquorice with turmeric and set aside.

Heat oil in a pan or wok and fry ginger for 1 minute. Add chicken and liquorice mixture and stir vigorously for 2 minutes.

Add spring onions, soy sauce, pepper and water. Bring to a brisk boil for 2 minutes, then dish out and serve hot with plain rice.

Black Tea with Liquorice and Apple Slices

Black tea is usually sold as 'Iron Goddess of Mercy' tea — *tie guan yin* in Mandarin or *teet goon yum* in Cantonese. When combined with liquorice and apple, the brew reduces phlegm, replenishes iron and improves metabolism. Tea leaves in general also contain essential amino acids and tannic acid that help aid digestion and lower blood pressure.

Preparation time: 10 minutes
Cooking time: 25 minutes
Serves 4

Water 750 ml (24 fl oz / 3 cups)

Liquorice root slivers 70 g (2¹/₂ oz), rinsed and drained

Apples 2, cored and sliced

Black tea leaves 1 Tbsp

Bring water to the boil in a pot. Add liquorice and apple and simmer for 10 minutes.

Remove pot from heat and strain contents into a teapot. Add tea leaves and infuse for 5 minutes. Serve warm.

Liquorice Tea with Ginger and Red Dates

This is a time-honoured recipe for a drink that helps to reduce phlegm and the effects of bronchitis, and also to calm anxiety and soothe nervous tension. The red dates give it a pleasant sweetness and may also be eaten.

Preparation time: 15 minutes
Cooking time: 45 minutes
Serves 4

Liquorice root slivers 140 g (4¹/₂ oz), rinsed and drained

Ginger 70 g (2¹/₂ oz), peeled and crushed

Dried Chinese red dates 10, pitted, rinsed and drained

Water 1 litre (32 fl oz / 4 cups)

Combine all ingredients in a pot. Bring to the boil and cook over high heat until liquid is reduced by half.

Remove liquorice and ginger to discard and serve warm with red dates. Drink tea twice a day if you have the symptoms mentioned above.

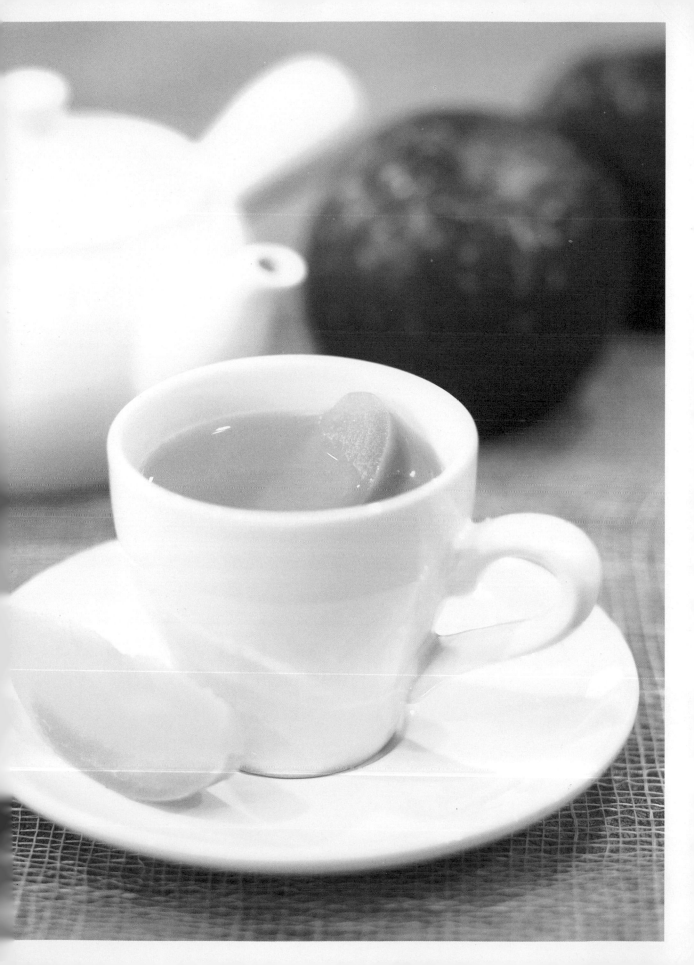

Longan

Common Longan
Mandarin Long yan
Cantonese Loong ngan
Botanical Euphoria longan arillus

The fresh longan, which literally means 'dragon's eye', is a seasonal fruit — each longan is about the size of a grape, with a greenish brown shell, and its translucent flesh, which encloses a round, dark brown seed, is sweet and succulent. A native of East Asia, the fruit is cultivated in China and Vietnam as well. It is never sold in its fresh state by Chinese herbalists, but in the dried form — either in their shells or as ready-shelled lumps of densely packed dried longan flesh. Much prized in China for its warming and tonic properties, the dried flesh is considered to be good for the spleen, heart, kidneys, lungs and mental faculties. It is also prescribed to treat nervous disorders, while the powdered kernel is used for styptic or astringent purposes. As a natural sweetener, it is a good substitute for sugar for a range of Chinese sweet soups and drinks — though not suitable for diabetics.

Longan, Gingko Nuts and Lotus Seeds

This is in the best tradition of the classic 'five-flavoured soup', or *ngo bee thng* in Hokkien, although a rather modified one using only three ingredients. Of the three, gingko nuts have the most medicinal value in addressing coughs, asthma and bladder problems.

Preparation time: 20 minutes
Cooking time: 15 minutes
Serves 4

Rock sugar 140 g (4 1/2 oz)

Screwpine (*pandan*) leaves 2, knotted

Water 1.5 litres (48 fl oz / 6 cups)

Precooked gingko nuts 30

Precooked lotus seeds 30

Dried longan flesh 80 g (3 oz), rinsed and drained

Combine rock sugar, screwpine leaves and water in a pot. Bring to the boil and simmer until sugar dissolves.

Add all other ingredients and simmer for 10–15 minutes, or until gingko nuts and lotus seeds are tender.

Remove screwpine leaves and discard. Serve hot or cold as a dessert.

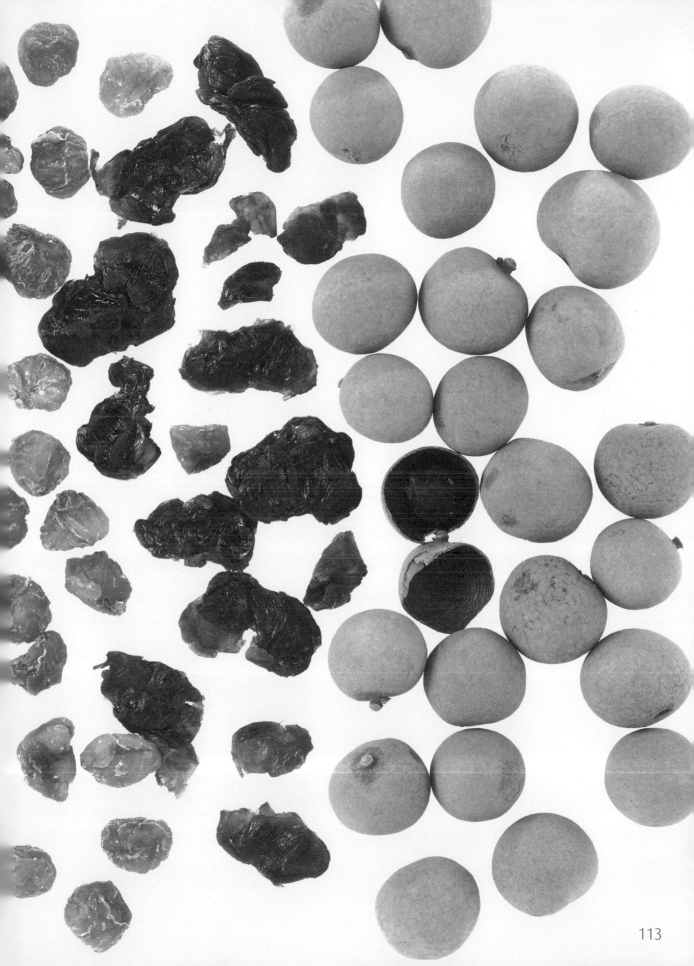

Longan and Mung Beans in Coconut Milk

This is an unusual dessert, eaten as a 'cooling' agent because of the mung beans. Coconut milk is very much my own infusion — as the sweet soup that echoes the soup my mother used to make for a late night snack. Always soak mung beans for a few hours, or preferably overnight as they then cook much faster.

Preparation time: 10 minutes (not including soaking overnight)
Cooking time: 1 hour
Serves 4

Mung (green) beans 100 g (3$^1/_2$ oz), rinsed clean, soaked for 2 hours and drained

Water 1 litre (32 fl oz / 4 cups)

Palm sugar 100 g (3$^1/_2$ oz)

Sugar 50 g (2 oz)

Salt $^1/_4$ tsp

Dried longan 150 g (5$^1/_3$ oz), rinsed and drained

Thick coconut milk 250 ml (8 fl oz / 1 cup)

Combine mung beans and water in a pot and bring to the boil over medium heat. Cover, reduce heat and simmer for 20–25 minutes, until mung beans are very soft.

Add both sugars, salt, and longan and simmer 5–10 minutes more, until beans are collapsing. Stir in coconut milk and cook until liquid is about to boil, then remove from heat. Serve warm or chilled.

Chicken with Mushrooms and Dried Longan

This is a light and delicious soup that has a subtle sweetness from the dried longan flesh.

Preparation time: 15 minutes
Cooking time: 40 minutes
Serves 4

Chicken breasts 2, skinned and cut into small dice

Chinese dried mushrooms 10, soaked or briefly boiled in water to soften, trimmed of hard stalks and caps quartered

Dried longan flesh 50 g (2 oz), rinsed and drained

Water 1 litre (32 fl oz / 4 cups)

Salt $^1/_2$ tsp

Ground black pepper $^1/_2$ tsp + extra for garnishing (optional)

Combine all ingredients in a pot and simmer for 40 minutes.

Ladle into individual serving bowls and sprinkle with pepper, if desired. Serve hot with rice and other dishes.

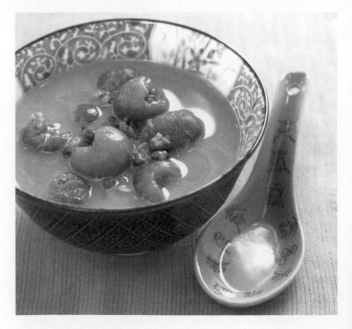

FROM LEFT TO RIGHT: Longan and Mung Beans in Coconut Milk (page 114), Chicken with Mushrooms and Dried Longan (page 114)

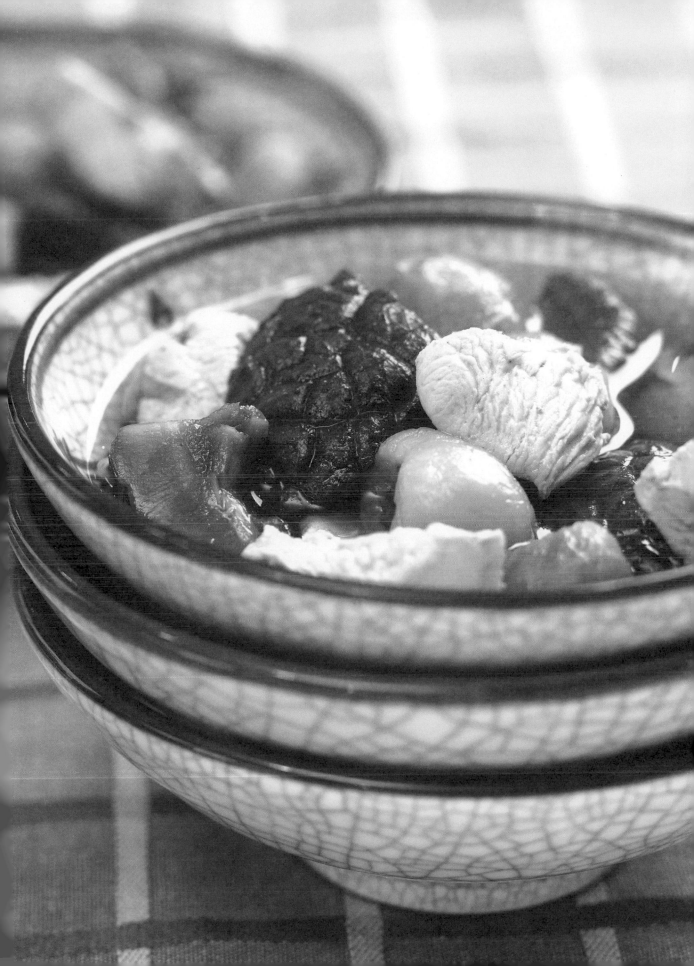

Lotus Root

Common Lotus root
Mandarin Lian ou
Cantonese Leen ngau
Botanical Nelumbo nucifera

This rhizome is from the same plant that gives us lotus seeds and is widely eaten either fresh, or dried in many Asian countries including China, Japan and Korea. Not strictly a herb, it is nonetheless regarded with a degree of respect in Chinese herbal cooking. The fresh form can be bought, covered with mud in wet markets or scrubbed clean and vacuum-packed in supermarkets. Lotus roots look like large tubers, each with numerous holes running down their lengths. They look like perforated pieces of marrow when sliced. Cooked with meat in soups and stews, it is believed to be good for the treatment of diabetes, irregular menstruation, constipation and stress. Younger rhizomes contain a starch that is similar to arrowroot and is boiled into a thin porridge to relieve diarrhoea and dysentery.

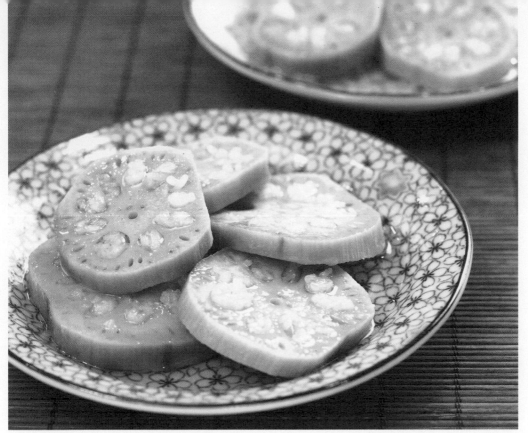

Lotus Root Stuffed with Glutinous Rice (page 117)

Lotus Root Stuffed with Glutinous Rice

This is a classic Chinese dessert known as *kuei hua t'ang lien ou* that may seem like a fiddly chore, but well worth the effort as a party piece. It reminds one of the cloying Teochew dessert of yam in sugar syrup called *oh nee*. What you will need is a chopstick or similar-sized prod to stuff rice into the lotus root cavities with.

Preparation time: 30 minutes
Cooking time: 45 minutes
Serves 4

Raw glutinous rice 75 g (2¹/₂ oz)

Lotus root 1, whole and in 2 segments, 600 g (1 lb 5 oz)

Sugar 70 g (2¹/₂ oz)

Sauce

Sugar 75 g (2¹/₂ oz)

Water 300 ml (10 fl oz /1¹/₄ cups)

Wash and cover rice with water to about 5 cm (2 in) above rice level. Soak for at least 2 hours.

Wash lotus root and scrape off outer skin thinly. Slice off about 2cm (1 in) from each end and retain. Wash and drain.

Drain excess water from rice and stuff rice into the hollows of lotus root. Replace sliced ends and secure with toothpicks. Blend sauce ingredients in a small pot.

Bring a large pot of water to the boil and cook lotus root for 20 minutes, or until soft enough to pierce with a skewer. Remove and cool.

Slice into 1-cm (¹/₂-in) rounds and arrange on a plate in a ring, with overlapping pieces. Sprinkle with sugar and cover with a piece of baking (greaseproof) paper. Steam for 30 minutes.

Boil sauce ingredients for 30 minutes, or until thick and glossy. Pour over lotus root slices and serve warm.

Lotus Seed

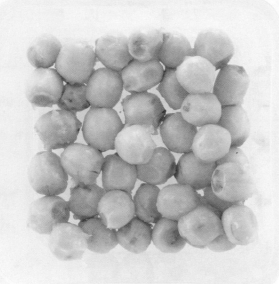

Common Lotus seed
Mandarin Lian zi
Cantonese Leen chi
Botanical Nelumbinis nucifera semen

Believed to be useful in promoting sleep, blood circulation and virility, lotus seeds are considered a neutral food, in that, it is neither 'warming' nor 'cooling'. They are also known to tonify the kidney and spleen, calm the heart, and stimulate sluggish appetites. Lotus seeds are believed to be good for treating diarrhoea as well. Because lotus seeds absorb the predominant flavour in a dish, they taste quite different when cooked with rock sugar in a dessert, or as part of savoury stuffing in a duck. Cooked lotus seeds have a texture not unlike boiled chestnuts, only more delicate.

Lotus Seed, Walnut and Red Date Tea

This tea is said to help prevent common colds, coughs and respiratory problems, strengthen kidney function and prevent constipation.

Preparation time: 10 minutes
Cooking time: 30 minutes
Serves 4

Precooked lotus seeds 40

Shelled whole walnuts 140 g
(5 oz), washed and drained

Dried Chinese red dates 140 g
(5 oz), pitted

Water 1 litre (32 fl oz / 4 cups)

Honey 4 Tbsp

Combine all ingredients in a pot and simmer for 30 minutes, then serve hot or chilled.

Pork Soup with Solomon's Seal and Lotus Seeds

This combination of herbs and pork is helpful in promoting good Qi balance, and healthy spleen and stomach functions.

Preparation time: 15 minutes
Cooking time: 1 hour
Serves 4

Lean pork 450 g (1 lb), washed and cut
into large chunks

Solomon's seal 15 g (1/2 oz),
rinsed and drained

Water 1 litre (32 fl oz / 4 cups)

Salt 2 tsp

Precooked lotus seeds 50 g (2 oz)

Combine pork, Solomon's seal and water in a pot and simmer for 45 minutes.

Add salt and lotus seeds and simmer for 15 minutes more. Serve hot.

Lotus Seed, Walnut and Red Date Tea (page 119)

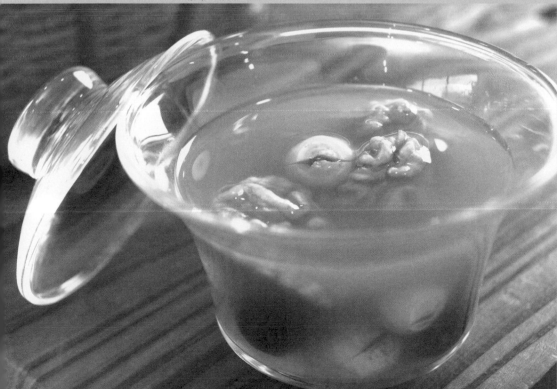

Mint

Garden variety mint leaves are much underrated. Of the 30-odd species in the mint family, peppermint and spearmint are probably the two best known varieties. Named after a nymph of Roman mythology, Minthe, the leaves of the plant have been used in the Mediterranean region for thousands of years and there are many references found in ancient Greek and Roman classics.

Mint is well known as a digestive aid, combatting dyspepsia and intestinal spasms. Mint is also used to treat fevers, headaches, coughs and sore throats. In Chinese herbal cooking, mint leaves are considered a 'cooling' food and are known as a digestive aid, useful in the treatment of irritable bowel syndrome. Mint also helps to regulate lung and liver functions, and reduce flatulence and colic. Catarrh problems may be treated with a regular intake of mint tea.

Common Mint
Mandarin Bo he
Cantonese Bok hor
Botanical Mentha arvensis

Minty New Potatoes

We take a broad leaf from the realm of European cuisine for this deliciously aromatic side offering. It is especially good with roast meats like lamb and chicken, but there is no reason why you cannot serve it as a light luncheon dish with all the minty promise.

Preparation time: 5 minutes
Cooking time: 25 minutes
Serves 4

New potatoes 500g (1 lb 1½ oz)

Fresh mint leaves 30 g (1 oz)

Salt 1 tsp

Olive oil 2 Tbsp

Freshly ground black pepper 1 tsp

Wash and scrub new potatoes but do not remove skins as they contain much of the nutrients and make good roughage as well.

Place in steamer and cook for 25 minutes until done but not mushy.

Chop mint leaves finely. Place potatoes in a salad bowl and toss with all seasonings and mint. Serve slightly chilled or warm as taste dictates.

Treatments

Bottles of **mint oil rub** of various brands are readily available at Chinese medicinal shops and are commonly prescribed for treating rheumatism as well as minor muscle cramps.

FROM LEFT TO RIGHT: Minty New Potatoes (page 121), Grilled Chicken with Mint, Mustard and Lime (page 122)

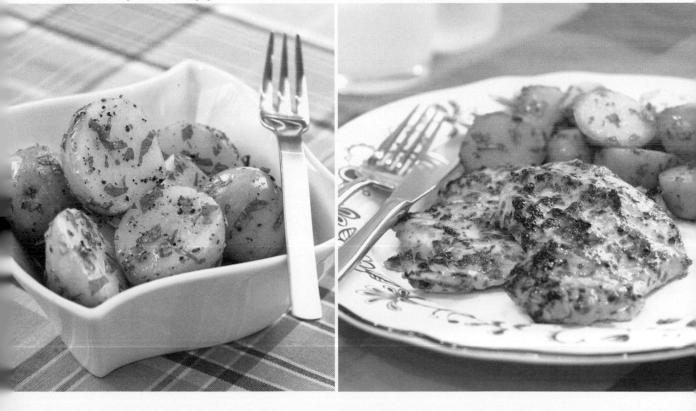

Grilled Chicken with Mint, Mustard and Lime

Mustard is often dismissed as a mere dip but really has spicy promise as a marinade. In this case, it is perfectly compatible with mint.

Preparation time: 10 minutes
Cooking time: 30 minutes
Serves 4

Chicken breasts 4, about 250 g (9 oz) each

Fresh mint leaves 30 g (1 oz), washed and drained

Yellow mustard 2 Tbsp

Lime juice 2 Tbsp

Salt 1 tsp

Sugar 2 tsp

Olive oil for basting 2 Tbsp

Halve each breast lengthways to make slightly thinner escalopes. Tenderise with the blunt edge of a cleaver.

Finely chop or grind mint leaves. Blend with mustard, lime juice, salt and sugar to make a marinade. Marinate chicken for an hour or so.

Place chicken on a grill pan and cook for 10 minutes on each side. Baste with a little olive oil.

When chicken is slightly charred around the edges, they should be done. Serve hot with Minty New Potatoes (see recipe on page 121).

Mint Tea with Honey and Red Dates

Preparation time: 5 minutes
Cooking time: 20 minutes
Serves 4

Water 600 ml (20 fl oz / 2¹/₂ cups)

Fresh mint leaves 30 g (1 oz), washed and drained

Dried Chinese red dates 10, pitted, rinsed and drained

Honey 2 Tbsp

Bring water to the boil in a pot. Add mint leaves and dates and simmer for 5 minutes.

Remove from heat, cover pot and leave to steep for 10 minutes.

Add honey and stir to incorporate flavours. Remove and discard mint leaves. Serve hot.

Treatment: Mint Oil Rub for Rheumatism (page 121)

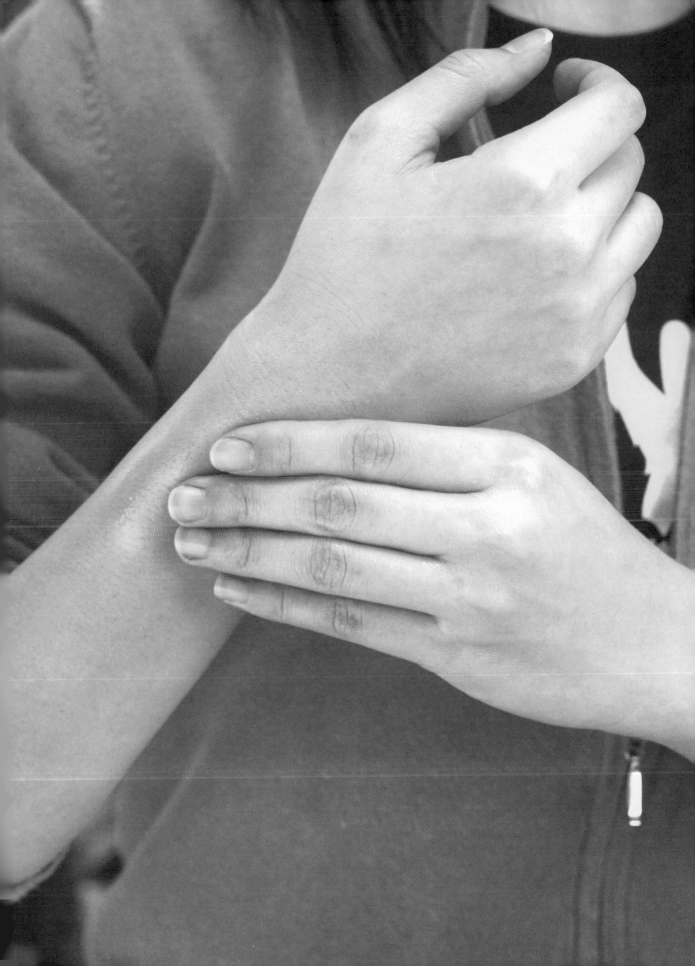

Myrrh

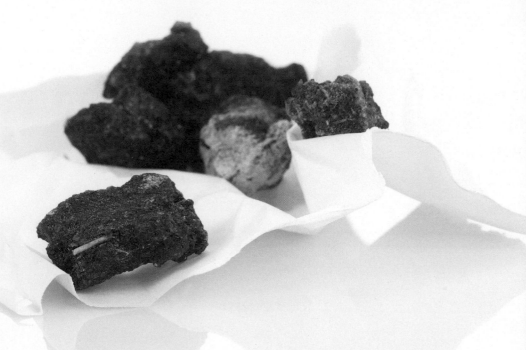

Common Myrrh
Mandarin Mo yao
Cantonese Mood yuk
Botanical Commiphora molmol, Commiphora myrrha

Myrrh resin looks like small, uneven brown pebbles. Truly a herbalist's cleansing agent, myrrh, with its anti-fungal, astringent and antiseptic properties that counter poisons, can be used to make a very soothing mouthwash. When added to soups and stews, the dishes become effective detoxifying agents.

Rarely taken orally, myrrh is, however, considered safe as a stabiliser and fragrance in cosmetics, as well as a flavouring in beverages. A neutral herb that influences the heart, liver and spleen functions, it also helps to activate sluggish blood flow and dispel blood clots. Myrrh is commonly used as a natural painkiller and for the treatment of irregular menstruation. It can also be externally applied in poultices to treat chronic sores and lesions from physical injuries.

Mutton with Chinese Angelica and Myrrh (page 126)

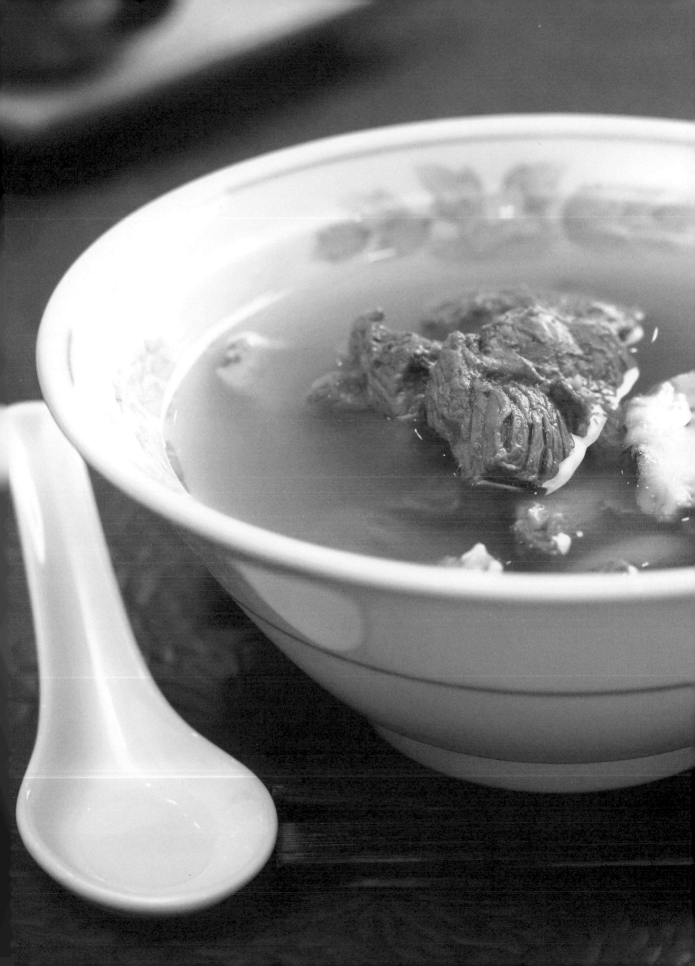

Myrrh and Clove Lemon Tea

On a cold day, this is a very comforting drink that also helps to detoxify the body.

Preparation time: 15 minutes
Cooking time: 10 minutes
Serves 4

Water 800 ml (26 fl oz / 3¹/₄ cups)

Myrrh 15 g (¹/₂ oz), rinsed and drained

Cloves 6

Ordinary tea bags 2

Lemon 1, juice squeezed

Honey (optional)

Bring water to the boil in a pot. Add myrrh and cloves and simmer for 10 minutes, then strain into a clean pot.

Return liquid to the boil, then switch off heat and immediately lower in tea bags to steep, covered, for 5 minutes.

Add lemon juice to tea before serving hot. Drizzle a little honey over, if desired.

Mutton with Chinese Angelica and Myrrh

Preparation time: 20 minutes
Cooking time: 2 hours
Serves 4

Water 1.5 litres (48 fl oz / 6 cups)

Mutton on the bone 1 kg (2 lb 3 oz), cleaned and cut into chunks

Chinese angelica 20 g (²/₃ oz), rinsed and drained

Myrrh 30 g (1 oz), rinsed and drained

Salt 2 tsp

Sugar 1 tsp

Ground black pepper 1 tsp

Chinese cooking wine (**shao hsing**) 4 Tbsp

Bring water to the boil in a pot. Add all remaining ingredients, except Chinese cooking wine. Simmer, covered, for 2 hours or until mutton falls off the bone.

Add Chinese wine in the last 5 minutes of cooking. Serve with rice and other dishes.

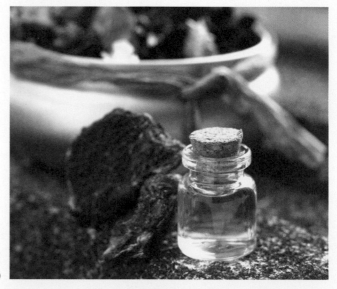

Aromatherapy: Myrrh Essential Oil (page 126)

Treatments
Myrrh has been used for centuries as an embalming ingredient and its tincture is very effective in treating chronic skin sores and lesions from injuries and athlete's foot.

Aromatherapy
Myrrh essential oil used in an aromatherapy burner is very uplifting. Its sweet, warm and slightly bitter aroma is invigorating.

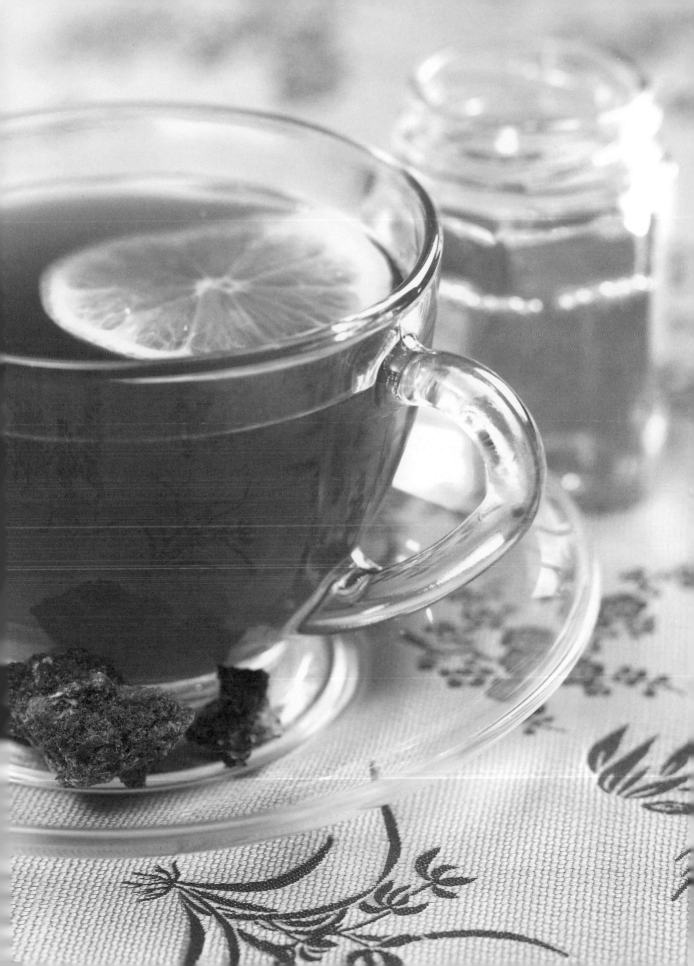

Nutmeg

Common Nutmeg
Mandarin Rou dou kou
Cantonese Yuk dau kau
Botanical Myristica fragrans

Native to the Moluccas and widely grown today in Indonesia, India and Malaysia, the nutmeg fruit is peach-like in appearance. When the outer husk is removed, the bright red lacy aril or fruit fibre is known as mace. Both mace and nutmeg are sold dried or powdered. In Chinese herbalism, nutmeg is used for regulating the large intestine, spleen and stomach functions. It is also good for preventing diarrhoea and is commonly used to dispel wind, and treat abdominal pain, vomitting and nausea as well as sluggish appetite.

Grilled Fish with Nutmeg, Cumin and Coriander (page 130)

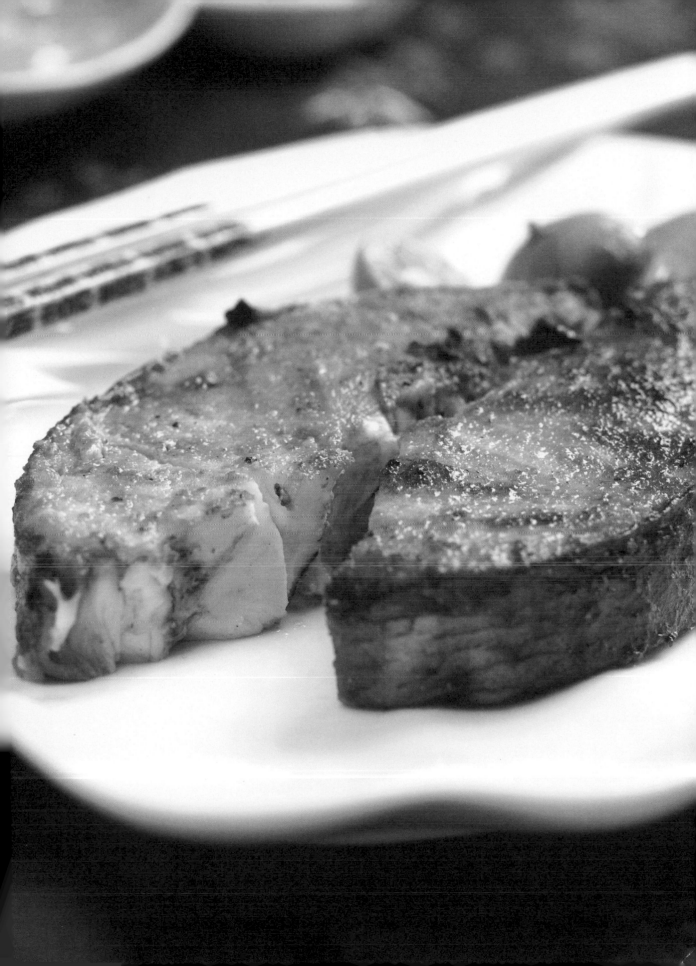

Chicken Soup with Nutmeg and Cloves

This is a take on the Indonesian *soto* soup, but with more efficacious promise from nutmeg and cloves.

Preparation time: 20 minutes
Cooking time: 30 minutes
Serves 4

Water 1 litre (32 fl oz / 4 cups)

Chicken breast 200 g (7 oz), cut into 1-cm (^{1}/$_2$-in) dice

Potatoes 120 g (4^1/$_2$ oz), peeled and cut into 1-cm (^{1}/$_2$-in) dice

Carrots 100 g (3^1/$_2$ oz), peeled and cut into 1-cm (^{1}/$_2$-in) dice

Nutmeg seed 10 g (^{1}/$_3$ oz)

Cloves 10

Light soy sauce 1 Tbsp

Lime juice 1 Tbsp

Ground black pepper 1 tsp

Freshly chopped coriander leaves (cilantro) 2 Tbsp

Bring water to the boil, then add chicken, potatoes and carrots. Simmer over medium heat for 25 minutes.

Add nutmeg, cloves, soy sauce, lime juice and pepper. Simmer for another 5 minutes. Remove from heat. Serve hot, garnished with coriander.

Grilled Fish with Nutmeg, Cumin and Coriander

This is a marvellous way to give ordinary fish a great lift, especially for a barbecue. Ground nutmeg is best for the marinade.

Preparation time: 10 minutes
Cooking time: 20 minutes
Serves 4

Threadfin (*ikan kurau*) 600 g (1 lb 5 oz)

Ground nutmeg 1 tsp

Cumin powder 1 Tbsp

Coriander powder 1 Tbsp

Salt 2 tsp

Sugar 1 tsp

Vegetable oil 2 Tbsp + more for basting

Kalamansi lime 1–2, halved

Clean and gut fish, then cut into large steaks, or leave whole, if desired.

Blend all other ingredients well and rub fish all over. Leave for 10 minutes.

Heat a charcoal burner and barbecue or grill fish for 4–5 minutes on each side, until golden brown and cooked. Baste with a little more oil, if required.

Serve hot with cut limes on the side, and squeeze some lime juice over fish before serving with rice and other dishes.

Note: Bruise a stalk of lemon grass at the root end to make a rough brush. Dip in oil and baste fish for a lovely citrus tang.

Treatments

To make a **massage oil for rheumatism and minor aches**, mix 5 drops of nutmeg essential oil with an equal amount of a base oil such as sweet almond oil, and gently rub onto the affected area topically.

Aromatherapy

For a relaxing bath, apply about 3 drops of nutmeg essential oil in a filled bathtub, while 3 drops of nutmeg essential oil mixed with 6 drops of any base oil can be heated in an aromatherapy burner for a soothing scent.

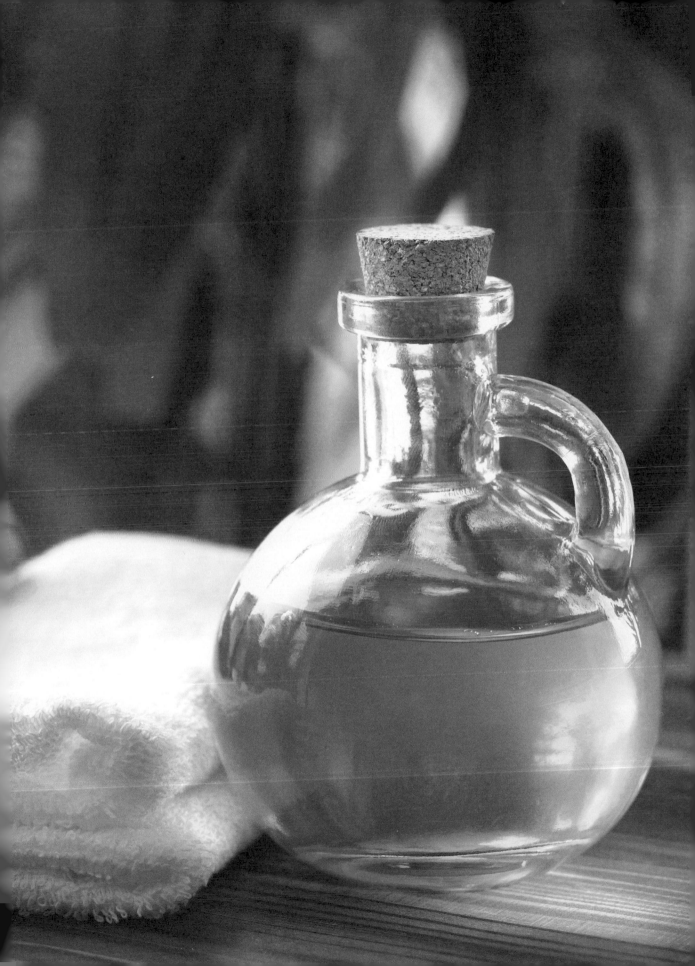

Common Pennywort, Asiatic pennywort
Mandarin Ji xue cao, Beng da wan,
Lei gong gen
Botanical Centella asiatica

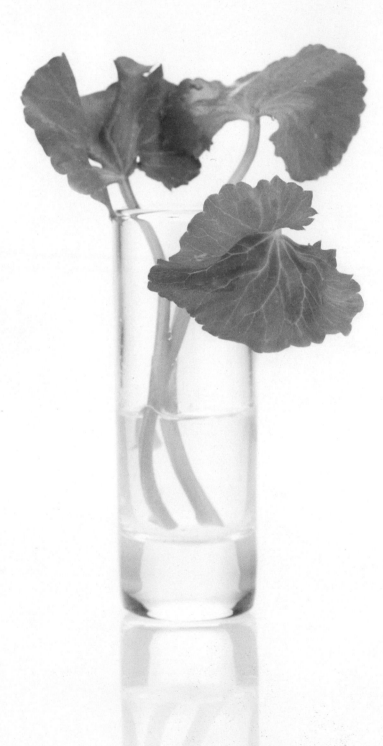

Also known as Asiatic pennywort, Indian pennywort, *daun pegaga* in Malay, or most famously as *gotu kola*, its Singhalese name, this most curious leaf stirs up many memories of my younger days, when my grandmother's backyard was a treasure trove of herbal culinary gems — their medicinal value, too, never overlooked.

My mother called it *hum kuck chao*, or 'scallop-shell leaf' in Teochew, on account of it being shaped so. Used liberally by Indian, Malay, Thai, Vietnamese and Nonya or Straits Chinese cooks, in salads and *ulam* (herb-based) meals, pennywort has long been associated with herbal brews. It is a veritable powerhouse leaf that I often use, now that it is regularly imported into Europe from Thailand.

The herb has anti-oxidant, anti-bacterial, anti-viral and anti-inflammatory qualities and is reputed to be effective over a wide range of applications. These include improving blood circulation, digestion, memory and longevity, as well as healing all manner of skin ailments, from burns to psoriasis.

Pennywort Salad

This was one of my grandmother's favourite, and she always had a pot of it growing in her backyard. There is little cooking involved apart from toasting the dried shrimp paste.

Preparation time: 15 minutes
Cooking time: 5 minutes
Serves 4

Indian pennywort 350 g (12 oz), washed and drained

Dressing

Red chillies 3–6, to taste

Dried shrimp paste (*belacan*) 1 Tbsp, toasted

Garlic 2 cloves, peeled

Dried prawns (shrimps) 100 g (3¹/₂ oz), soaked in hot water to soften, then drained and coarsely ground

Lime juice 3 Tbsp

Sugar 1 Tbsp

Cut and discard roots of pennywort, if any, and trim each stem to about 5 cm (2 in) from the leaf. Place leaves in a serving bowl and set aside.

Prepare dressing. Finely grind chillies, shrimp paste and garlic together using a blender (processor), or mortar and pestle. Transfer to a bowl, then add dried prawns, lime juice and sugar. Mix well.

Add desired amount of dressing to pennywort leaves. Toss until well-mixed and serve.

Note: If you find the bitterness of pennywort too strong, modify the salad by halving the amount of pennywort used and replacing with other salad leaves such as rocket (arugula) or iceberg lettuce, or other Asian herbs like polygonum (laksa) leaves, coriander leaves (cilantro) or even bean sprouts.

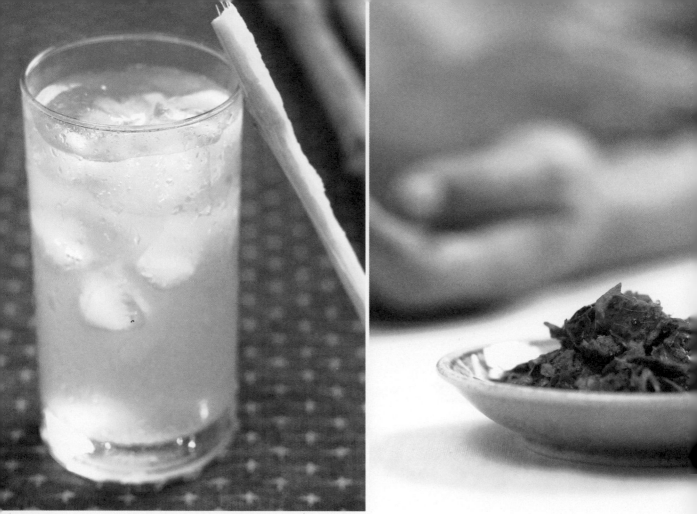

FROM LEFT TO RIGHT: Pennywort Drink with Sugar Cane (page 134), Treatment: Poultice for Minor Burns and Wounds (page 134), Pennywort Salad (page 133)

Pennywort Drink with Sugar Cane

Indians are fond of chilled pennywort drinks as it cools down the system, especially after fish head curry! This is a more way of preparing a 'yin' or 'cooling' drink with the leaf.

Preparation time: 10 minutes
Cooking time: 35 minutes
Serves 4

Pennywort 350 g (11 oz), washed and drained

Sugar cane 3 sticks, each about 30-cm (12-in) long, washed well and trimmed of discoloured parts

Rock sugar 75 g (2 1/2 oz)

Water 1.5 litres (48 fl oz / 6 cups)

Cut away pennywort roots and trim each stem to about 5 cm (2-in) from the leaf. Set aside.

Bruise sugar cane and cut into pieces short enough to fit into a large pot. Halve pieces lengthwise. Combine sugar cane, rock sugar and water. Bring to the boil, cover and simmer over medium-low heat for 30 minutes.

Add pennywort and simmer 5 minutes more, then strain and serve warm or chilled.

Treatments

My herbalist adviser, Dr. Geng, says a poultice of ground pennywort leaves can be applied onto skin that has psoriasis to soothe itchiness and aid healing. To make a **poultice for minor burns and wounds**, simply crush pennywort leaves and apply on the affected area. You can also mix about 10 crushed leaves with 1 Tbsp aloe vera gel for better staying power. Apply several times a day, and for about an hour each time.

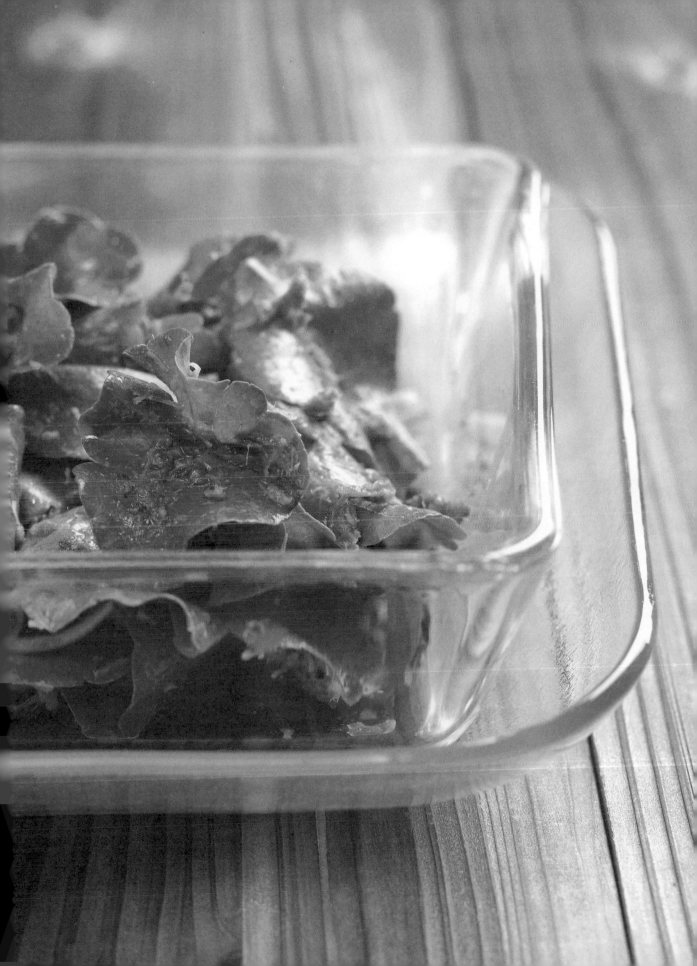

Pumpkin Seed

Common Pumpkin seed
Mandarin Nan gua zi
Cantonese Nahm gwa chi

Pumpkin seeds contain several major groups of active constituents: essential fatty acids, amino acids, carbohydrates and minerals. The oil has been used in combination with saw palmetto to effectively reduce symptoms of enlarged prostrates. Other tests have also shown that pumpkin seed extracts can improve the functions of the bladder and urethra.

Scientific research has indicated that the constituent called curcurbitin in pumpkin seeds appears to have anti-parasitic activity and can help resolve tapeworm infestations. Pumpkin seeds are also used for healing burns and wounds, easing the digestion of carbohydrates, enhancing the growth and development of the reproductive and sex organs, as well as improving phosphorus and protein metabolism. Scientific trials in Thailand have reportedly found that eating pumpkin seeds as a snack can help prevent the most common type of kidney stones; the seeds appear to reduce the levels of substances that promote stone formation in the urine, and increase levels of substances that inhibit stone formation at the same time.

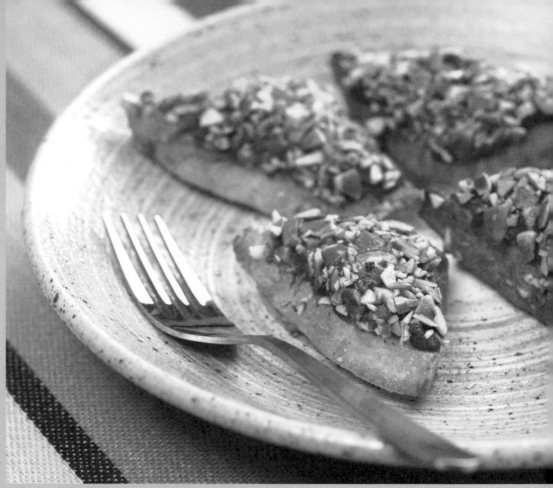

Pumpkins Seeds and Minced Pork on Toasts (page 138)

Pumpkin Seeds and Minced Pork on Toasts

It is more a snack food item than a culinary mainstay, but pumpkin seeds can be as versatile as sesame seeds. Eat a handful a day, and you are less likely to suffer from prostrate problems.

Preparation time: 15 minutes
Cooking time: 10 minutes
Serves 4

White bread 4 slices, crusts removed and cut into 4 triangles each

Eggs 2, lightly beaten

Minced pork 120 g (4^1/$_2$ oz), mixed with 1 tsp salt

Pumpkin seeds 100 g (3^1/$_2$ oz), finely ground using a mortar and pestle

Cooking oil for deep-frying

With each bread triangle, first brush on some beaten egg, then top with ^{1}/$_2$ Tbsp minced pork and spread it out evenly.

Dip bread, pork side down, into ground pumpkin seeds and shake off any excess. Repeat until ingredients are used up.

Deep-fry filled bread pieces in hot oil until golden brown, then drain on paper towels. Serve as a snack.

Treatments
Pumpkin seed oil is derived from Styrian pumpkins that contain dark green seeds with no outer shells. As a result, the seeds are easily processed into oil. Pumpkin seeds contain vitamins A, B1, B2, B6, C, D, E, and K, as well as calcium and magnesium. The oil also contains over 60 percent of unsaturated fatty acid and is rich in vegetable protein. Recent medical research has also shown that they help to regulate cholesterol levels. You can buy pumpkin seed tablets that are usually a blend with saw palmetto and zinc to treat prostrate problems.

Bean and Sweetcorn Salad with Pumpkin Seeds and Oil

Pumpkin seed oil, because of its nutritional properties and nutty flavour, is now widely used by Mediterranean chefs in salads and as a frying agent. This is a fairly simple salad using both the seeds and the oil for healthy measure. Use canned beans as they require no cooking.

Preparation time: 15 minutes
Cooking time: 10 minutes
Serves 4

Canned flageolet white beans
100 g (3¹/₂ oz), drained

Canned red kidney beans
100 g (3¹/₂ oz), drained

Canned sweetcorn kernels
100 g (3¹/₂ oz), drained

Pumpkin seeds 80 g (3 oz)

Lettuce leaves (optional)

Dressing

Pumpkin seed oil 4 Tbsp

Wine vinegar 2 Tbsp

Sugar 1 tsp

Salt 1 tsp

Combine both beans and sweetcorn in a salad bowl and set aside.

Combine all dressing ingredients in a bottle, seal and shake well, or stir them together in a bowl until well-blended.

Toss bean salad with dressing and pumpkin seeds until evenly mixed. Serve on individual plates lined with lettuce leaves, if desired.

Bean and Sweetcorn Salad with Pumpkin Seeds and Oil (page 139)

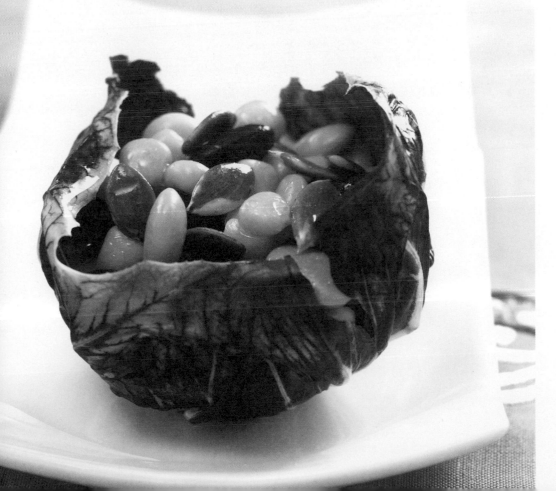

139

Reshi Mushroom

Common Reshi mushroom, Ganoderma mushroom
Mandarin Ling zhi
Cantonese Leng chi
Botanical Ganoderma lucidum

Going by the Chinese name of *ling zhi*, this fungus has been a herbal mainstay for more than 4,000 years in China, its legend bordering on the mystical. Its Chinese name means 'herb of spiritual potency' and was much sought after by mountain sages and emperors alike. The iconic Chinese imagery, is that of a deer feeding on a *ling zhi* mushroom beside the God of Longevity.

A polypore mushroom that is soft when fresh, corky, and flat with a red-varnished cap, it has white to dull brown pores underneath. Unlike other mushrooms, polypores have no gills on their underside, and release their spores through pores; hence, the term, 'polypore'. It is believed that much of the curative powers of the mushroom comes from its spores, which are available only on a cyclical basis, and therefore not easy to harvest.

In modern applications and other herbal uses, *ling zhi*'s therapeutic value is very much sought after in anti-cancer treatments. It is also a panacea for cardiac problems, severe allergies, liver conditions and regulating cholesterol levels. In fact, the Reishi mushroom has become so well-known that it has been added to the American Herbal Pharmacopoeia and Therapeutic Compendium. Most Chinese herbalists sell Reishi mushrooms whole and dried, sliced and dried, and also in tablet or powder form.

Duck Soup with Reishi Mushrooms and Gingko Nuts

When well-done, duck is ambrosial despite its reputation for being strong-smelling. As it is a fatty bird, skinning the bird alleviates this to a large degree.

Preparation time: 20 minutes
Cooking time: 2 hours
Serves 4

Duck 1, about 1.5 kg (3 lb 4¹/₂ oz)
Reishi mushroom slices 30 g (1 oz), rinsed and drained
Tangerine peel 10 g (¹/₃ oz)
Water 2 litres (64 fl oz / 8 cups)
Precooked gingko nuts 40
Salt 2 tsp
Ground black pepper 1 tsp

Clean duck thoroughly and skin, removing every bit of blood and entrails. Cut into 8 joints, then rub with plenty of salt. Rinse thoroughly and drain well.

Combine duck, Reishi mushroom slices, tangerine peel and water in a pot with a snug-fitting lid. Cover pot and simmer for about 1 hour 40 minutes, checking water level every now and then.

Add gingko nuts, salt and pepper, then simmer for about 20 minutes more. Serve with rice and other dishes.

Note: If using a pressure cooker, simmer over medium heat for 45 minutes, then remove from heat and release pressure to add gingko nuts, salt and pepper. After that, cook, uncovered, for 20 minutes. If soup is still oily at the end of cooking, allow to cool and skim off layer of duck fat with a spoon.

Chicken Soup with Reishi Mushrooms and Wolfberries

This soup is particularly good for people who suffer from severe allergies and are recovering from them.

Preparation time: 20 minutes
Cooking time: 1 hour
Serves 4

Chicken 1, about 1.5 kg (3 lb 4¹/₂ oz) cleaned, skinned and quartered

Reishi mushroom slices 30 g (1 oz), rinsed and drained

Chinese wolfberries 1 Tbsp, rinsed and drained

Water 1.5 litres (48 fl oz / 6 cups)

Salt 2 tsp

Combine all ingredients in a pot and simmer over medium heat for 1 hour.

Serve hot at the beginning of a meal.

Note: Traditionally, the chicken is not eaten, but that is not to say that it is inedible. It will taste rather bland, however, so serve with a side dip of light soy sauce, if you intend to eat it.

Treatments

Ling zhi capsules are now readily available at many Chinese medicinal shops, and are sold as a health supplement for the maintenance of general health and the strengthening of the body's immune system. The capsules are reportedly useful for the nourishment of body organs including the liver, heart, lungs and kidneys as well. They can also be taken for the treatment of various ailments including insomnia, asthma and sluggish appetite, and are recommended for cancer patients undergoing chemotherapy.

FROM LEFT TO RIGHT: Treatment: Ling Zhi Capsules for Good Health (page 142), Chicken Soup with Reishi Mushrooms and Wolfberries (page 142)

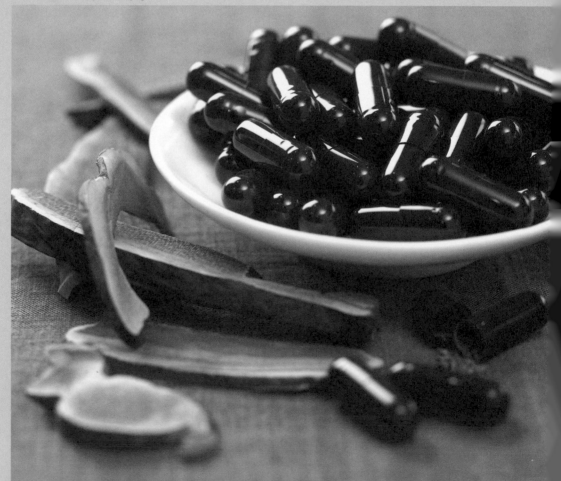

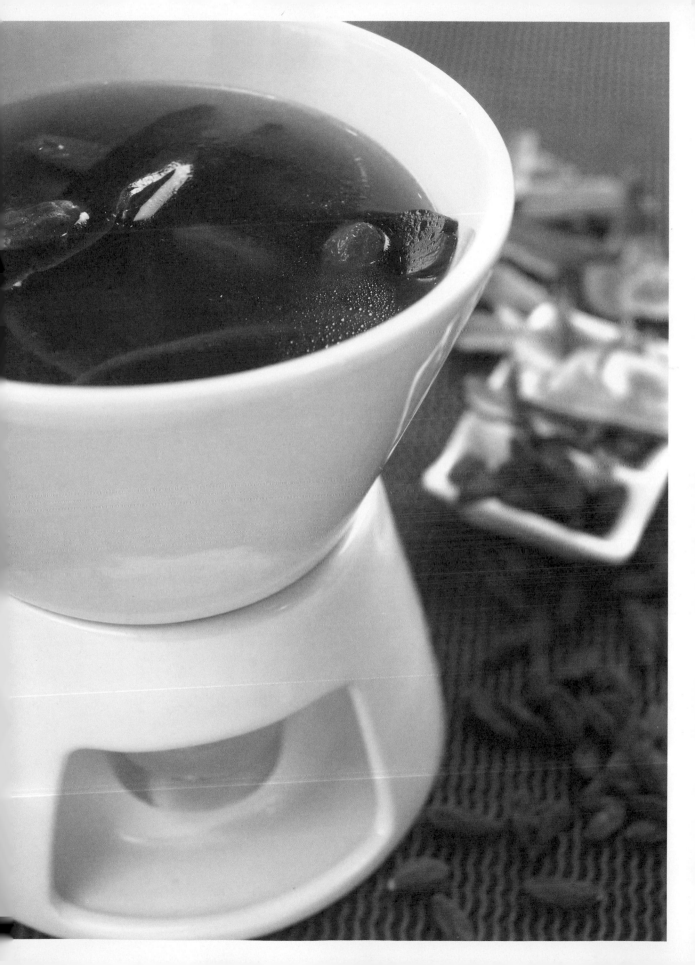

Saffron

Saffron may be famous for its culinary ingenuity to transform mundane rice to glorious, golden heights in Indian cuisine, but it is also much touted in Indian Ayurvedic medicine for its calming effect. Saffron threads are the hand-picked stigmas of the saffron flowers that grow in the mountainous areas of northern China, the Himalayas and most famously, in Kashmir. It has antiseptic action, is slightly laxative and diuretic.

TCM references to saffron, however, also include the safflower or bastard saffron (*carthamus tinctorius*) as both varieties are commonly called *hong hua* in Mandarin which simply means 'red flower'. Saffron is used for the treatment of heart, liver and bladder functions. Believed to dispel blood stagnation, reduce pain and uterine bleeding, the spice is traditionally used during childbirth.

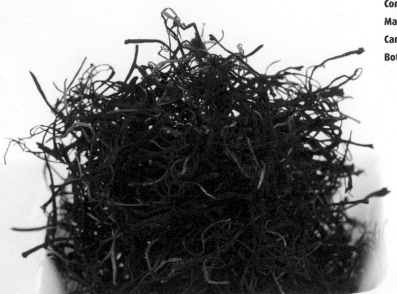

Common Saffron
Mandarin Xi zang hong hua
Cantonese Sai jong hong fah
Botanical Crocus sativus

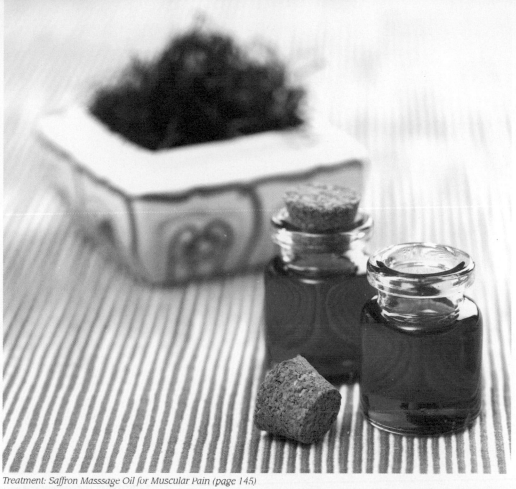

Treatment: Saffron Masssage Oil for Muscular Pain (page 145)

Treatments

Often labelled as 'Tibetan Saffron Flower Oil' or ' Red Flower Oil', small bottles of **saffron massage oil for muscular pain** can be purchased at many Chinese medicinal shops. It is effective in relieving backache, sciatica and rheumatic pain, as well as strains and bruises associated with minor sports injuries or stiffness after physical exercises. To use, simply apply a few drops on the affected areas and massage well into the skin.

Sichuan Soup

This spicy soup is particularly good for new mothers as it is believed to heal childbirth pains and regulate menstrual cycles.

Preparation time: 20 minutes
Cooking time: 45 minutes
Serves 4

Chicken 1, about 1.5 kg (3 lb 4 ½ oz), cleaned, skinned and cut into large joints

Saffron 1 tsp

Sichuan peppercorns 2 tsp

Water 1.5 litres (48 fl oz / 6 cups)

Salt 2 tsp

Chopped spring onions (scallions) 2 Tbsp

Ground black pepper to taste

Combine chicken, saffron, Sichuan peppercorns, water and salt in a pot. Simmer for 45 minutes or until chicken falls off the bone.

Remove chicken pieces and cool before deboning and shredding the meat. Simmer soup over low heat to keep warm.

Return chicken to simmering soup and stir through. Heat for 1–2 minutes, then ladle into individual serving bowls.

Garnish with spring onions and a sprinkling of black pepper to taste. Serve hot with rice and other dishes, if desired.

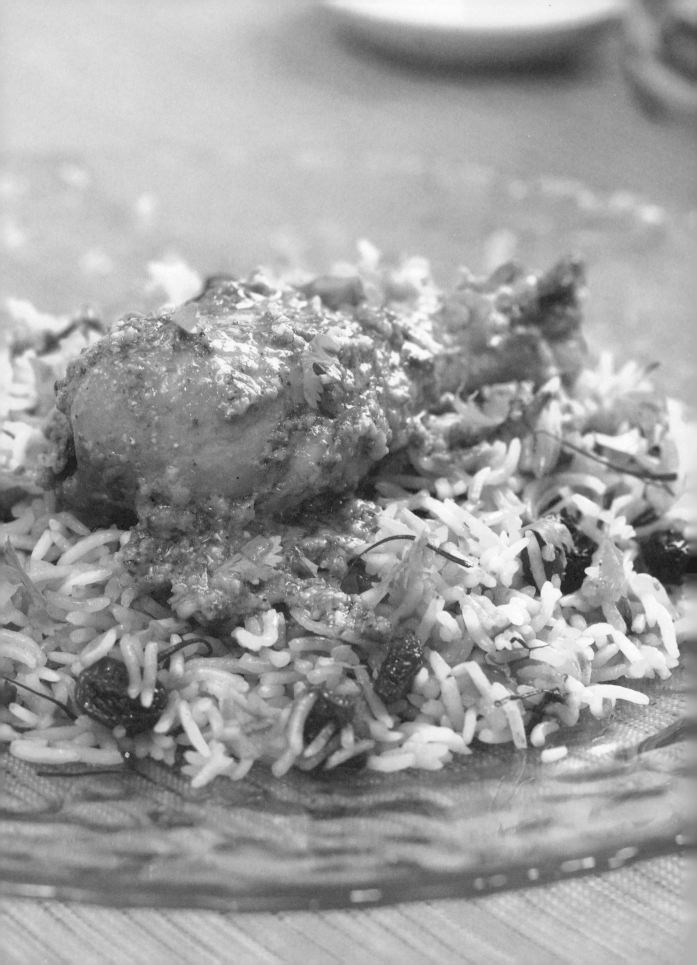

Saffron Rice with Biryani Chicken

In Tibet and India, saffron is attributed with aphrodisiac powers — so bring on the Biryani!

Preparation time: 35 minutes
Cooking time: 55 minutes
Serves 6

Coconut milk 500 ml (16 fl oz / 2 cups)

Evaporated milk 100 ml
(3¹/₃ fl oz / ³/₈ cup)

Ground almonds 4 Tbsp

Lime juice 2 Tbsp

Cooking oil 3 Tbsp

Cinnamon stick 1, 5-cm (2-in) long

Cardamom 8 pods

Green chillies 4, split lengthways
and seeded if desired

Chopped coriander leaves 4 Tbsp

Chicken legs 6, halved at the joints

Salt 2 tsp

Spice Paste

Garlic 6 cloves, peeled and left whole

Chopped ginger 2 Tbsp

Water 2 Tbsp

Coriander powder 1 Tbsp

Ground cumin 1 Tbsp

Ground fennel 2 tsp

Turmeric powder 1 tsp

Chilli powder 1 tsp

Ground black pepper 1 tsp

Saffron Rice

Cooking oil 2 Tbsp

Shallots 8, peeled and sliced

Basmati rice 450 g (1 lb),
washed, soaked for
at least 1 hour and drained

Water 1 litre (32 fl oz / 4 cups)

Salt 1 tsp

Raisins or sultanas 100 g (3¹/₂ oz)

Saffron 1 Tbsp, soaked in 4 Tbsp warm
water for 15 minutes

Rose water 1 Tbsp

Prepare spice paste. Blend (process) all ingredients together until smooth and set aside.

Mix coconut milk, evaporated milk, ground almonds and lime juice together. Set mixture aside for a few minutes to thicken slightly.

Heat oil in a wok or pan over medium-high heat. Add spice paste, cinnamon and cardamom and fry for 2 minutes, stirring constantly. Add green chillies and coriander and fry for 1 minute more, until fragrant.

Add chicken pieces and fry for 1 minute, stirring to mix thoroughly. Add milk mixture and salt and bring to the boil. Partially cover, reduce heat and simmer for 35–40 minutes, or until liquid has reduced to a thick gravy.

Prepare saffron rice. Heat oil in a pan over medium heat. Fry shallots until browned, 3–4 minutes. Add rice and stir gently but constantly for 2 minutes. Add water and salt, then transfer rice to a deep pot or rice cooker to finish cooking.

When rice is almost dry, with still a little moisture on top, stir in raisins or sultanas, then add saffron and soaking liquid, mixing well to form golden streaks in rice mixture. Cover and cook until rice grains are light and fluffy.

When rice is cooked, spread half the amount in a large heatproof (flameproof) casserole. Lift biryani chicken pieces from pot, leaving gravy behind and arrange them in a single layer on top of rice mixture. Top with remaining rice and sprinkle with rose water.

Cover tightly and bake in a preheated oven at 160°C (325°F) for 10 minutes, to let the flavours of rice and chicken meld together. Remove from oven and serve immediately.

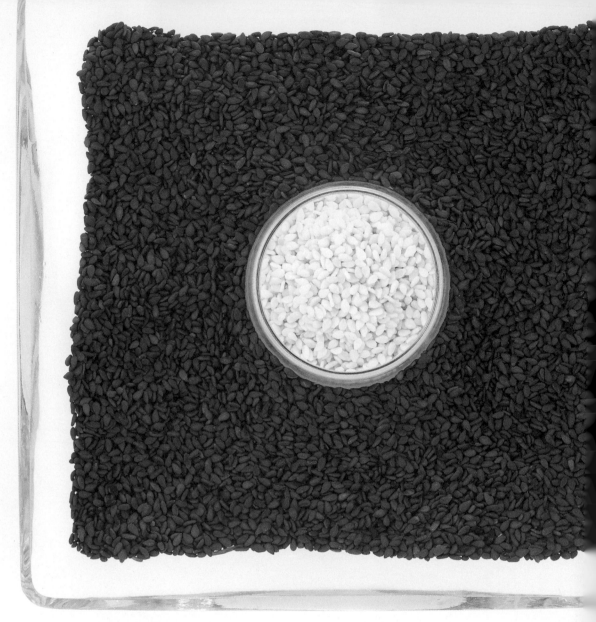

Sesame

Common Sesame
Mandarin Zhi ma
Cantonese Chi mah
Botanical Sesamum indicum

As a culinary ingredient, black sesame seeds make frequent appearances as a topping — sprinkled on top of dishes. While the common white variety is less known for their efficacious promise, black sesame seeds are used as a tonic to improve liver and kidney functions in TCM. They also help to nourish the blood, dispel wind and relieve 'dryness' of the body system as well as treat headaches and constipation.

Sesame Custard

A good friend cooked this most unusual dish for me, saying that it used to be the vegetarian mainstay of Buddhist monks in northern China. It requires a little work but is well worth the effort. It is almost like making bean curd but has nothing to do with soy beans.

Preparation time: 30 minutes
Cooking time: 25 minutes
Serves 4

White sesame seeds 200 g (7 oz)

Water 1 litre (32 fl oz / 4 cups)

Arrowroot flour 100 g (3½ oz), mixed with 150 ml (5 fl oz / ⅝ cup) water into a paste

Honey to taste (optional)

Combine sesame seeds and water in a blender (processor) and blend (process) into a fine paste.

Line a bowl with a piece of fine muslin cloth, then pour sesame paste over. Gather edges of cloth and squeeze gently to extract a milky smooth liquid.

Transfer sesame liquid to a non-stick or heavy-bottomed pot. Add arrowroot paste and bring to a slow simmer. Stir gently but continuously with a wooden spoon until mixture thickens and becomes glossy; it will bubble furiously, but do not stop stirring.

Remove from heat and pour into a deep dish or mould. Allow to cool and set, but do not refrigerate.

Cut into squares, drizzle honey over and serve as a dessert, if desired. Alternatively, use as you would bean curd in savoury dishes.

Black Sesame Cream (page 150)

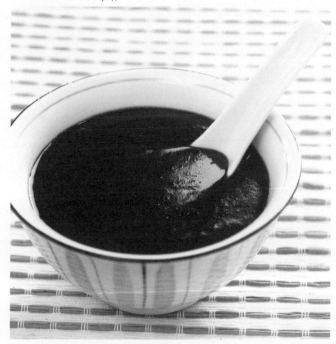

Black Sesame Cream

Cantonese-speakers know this classic dessert as *chi mah woo*. My local hawker of some four decades ago came along every evening like clockwork to sell this lovely dessert, and many a sustaining bowl was downed after late nights of mahjong.

Preparation time: 25 minutes
Cooking time: 25 minutes
Serves 4

Black sesame seeds 450 g (1 lb)

Water 800 ml (26 fl oz / 3 1/4 cups)

Sugar 200 g (7 oz) or more to taste

Arrowroot flour 3 Tbsp, mixed with 150 ml (5 fl oz / 5/8 cup) into a paste

Mix black sesame seeds with sufficient water to make a loose slurry. Pour into a blender (processor) and blend (process) into a fine paste, adding more water if necessary — this should take 2–4 minutes. Blend (process) at intervals, if your blender overheats.

Transfer paste to a pot, add remaining water and whisk until mixture is smooth. Bring to a slow boil over medium-low heat. Stir in sugar, then simmer, stirring continuously, for 25 minutes.

Add arrowroot paste and stir for 5–6 minutes more, until thickened. Taste and adjust with more sugar, if desired. Serve warm.

Note: It is best to use a high-powered blender (food processor) for grinding the sesame seeds with water, as they take a while to be reduced to a paste. Add only just enough water to keep the blades turning — if the mixture is too wet, the seeds will not be ground fine enough.

Sesame Chilli Dip

This is an excellent dip for fried foods or barbecued meats.

Preparation time: 15 minutes
Serves 4

Red chillies 6

Garlic 3 cloves, peeled and left whole

Chopped ginger 1 Tbsp

Fish sauce 3 Tbsp

Lime juice 2 Tbsp

Melted palm sugar 1 Tbsp

White sesame seeds 1 Tbsp

Chopped spring onions (scallions) 1 Tbsp

Finely grind chillies, garlic and ginger using a blender (processor), or mortar and pestle.

Transfer ground ingredients to a small bowl and mix in remaining ingredients. Serve as a dip for fried or barbecued foods.

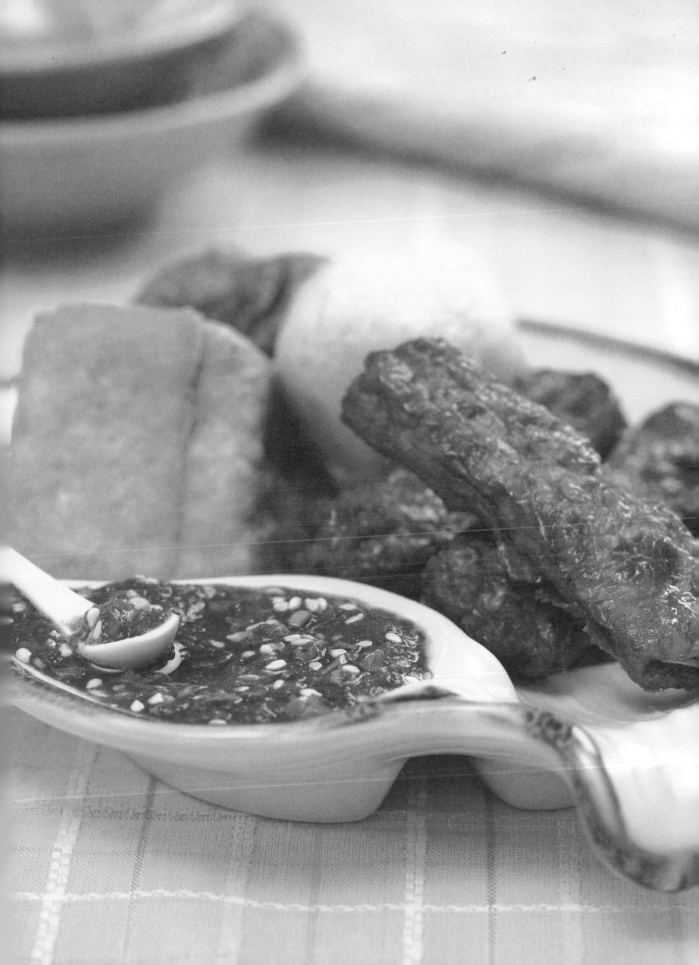

Sichuan Peppercorn

Common Sichuan peppercorn
Mandarin Chuan jiao
Cantonese Fu chiu
Botanical Zanthoxylum piperitum

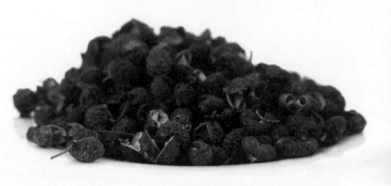

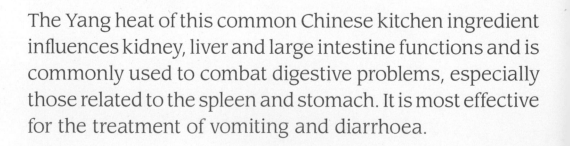

The Yang heat of this common Chinese kitchen ingredient influences kidney, liver and large intestine functions and is commonly used to combat digestive problems, especially those related to the spleen and stomach. It is most effective for the treatment of vomiting and diarrhoea.

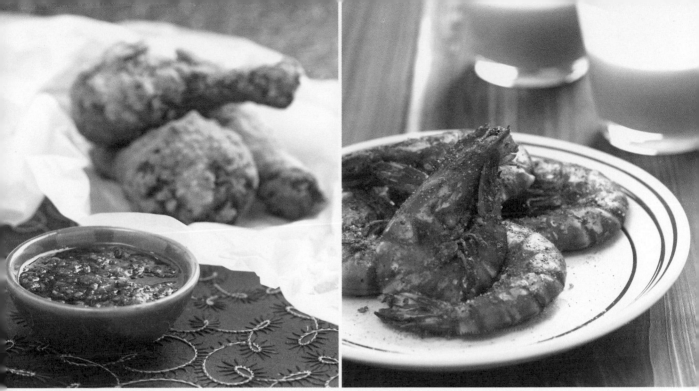

FROM LEFT TO RIGHT: Sichuan Pepper and Sesame Dip with Fried Chicken (page 153), Salt and Pepper Prawns (page 153)

Sichuan Pepper and Sesame Dip

This makes a delicious dip for fried foods and other barbecued meats.

Preparation time: 20 minutes
Serves 4

Sichuan peppercorns 1 Tbsp
Garlic 2 cloves, peeled and left whole
Chopped ginger 1 Tbsp
Sesame oil 2 Tbsp
Light soy sauce 1 Tbsp
Sugar 1 tsp

Grind peppercorns with garlic and ginger using a mortar and pestle.

Transfer mixture to a small bowl and stir in remaining ingredients until well-blended. Serve as a dip with fried foods or barbecued meats.

Salt and Pepper Prawns

This dish should never be cooked with shelled prawns as you get much less of the flavour.

Preparation time: 15 minutes
Cooking time: 10 minutes
Serves 4

Sichuan peppercorns 1 Tbsp
Salt 2 tsp
Cooking oil 3 Tbsp
Tiger prawns (shrimps) 16, washed, cleaned, trimmed and dried with paper towels
Sesame oil 2 Tbsp

Grind peppercorns until fine using a mortar and pestle, then mix in salt. Set aside.

Heat oil in a wok and flash-fry prawns until they turn slightly pink.

Add peppercorn mixture and stir-fry for 1 minute, then add sesame oil and stir-fry over high heat for 1–2 minutes, or until prawns are completely pink.

Dish out and serve immediately with rice and other dishes, if desired.

Roast Duck with Sichuan Pepper Sauce

Sichuan peppercorns, though basically similar in heat potential to regular peppercorns, have a pungent flavour that is reminiscent of liquorice. They are able to cut through a duck's oily richness to leave a warm, sweet flavour that is most enticing.

Preparation time: 25 minutes
Cooking time: 2 hours
Serves 4

Duck 1, about 2 kg (4 lb 6 oz), cleaned and trimmed of excess fat

Sichuan peppercorns 1 Tbsp

Garlic 3 cloves, peeled and left whole

Honey 2 Tbsp

Chinese cooking wine (shao hsing) 2 Tbsp

Bring a kettle of water to the boil and scald duck all over, including the inside, then hang up to dry overnight.

On the day of roasting, grind peppercorns and garlic together, using a mortar and pestle until very fine, then blend with honey and Chinese cooking wine.

Preheat oven at 220°C (440°F) for 20 minutes. Meanwhile, rub duck all over with peppercorn mixture and place on a roasting rack set over a baking pan.

Roast duck in preheated oven for 25 minutes, then reduce heat to 180°C (350°F), and continue to roast for 1 hour 30 minutes, or until cooked through.

To test for doneness, insert a metal skewer into the thickest part of the duck (between thigh and body). If liquid runs clear, the duck is done; its skin should be crispy. Cut into bite-sized pieces and serve hot with rice and other dishes, if desired.

Coriander and Cucumber Salad with Sichuan Pepper

My neighbours from Hubei often prepare this spicy salad whenever they invite me to dinner. It is a much-loved salad in their hometown.

Preparation time: 20 minutes
Serves 4

Coriander leaves (cilantro) 150 g (5 1/3 oz), washed, drained and roughly shredded

Cucumber 1, peeled, cored and grated into coarse shreds, then thoroughly washed and drained

Toasted white sesame seeds 2 Tbsp

Dressing

Sichuan peppercorns 2 tsp

Green chillies 4, seeded, if desired, and sliced

Garlic 2 cloves, peeled and left whole

Vegetable oil 2 Tbsp

Sugar 1 Tbsp

Rice vinegar 2 Tbsp

Prepare dressing. Grind Sichuan peppercorns, green chillies and garlic together until fine, using a mortar and pestle. Stir in oil, sugar and rice vinegar until well-blended.

Combine coriander and cucumber in a salad bowl and toss with dressing until evenly mixed. Serve, garnished with sesame seeds.

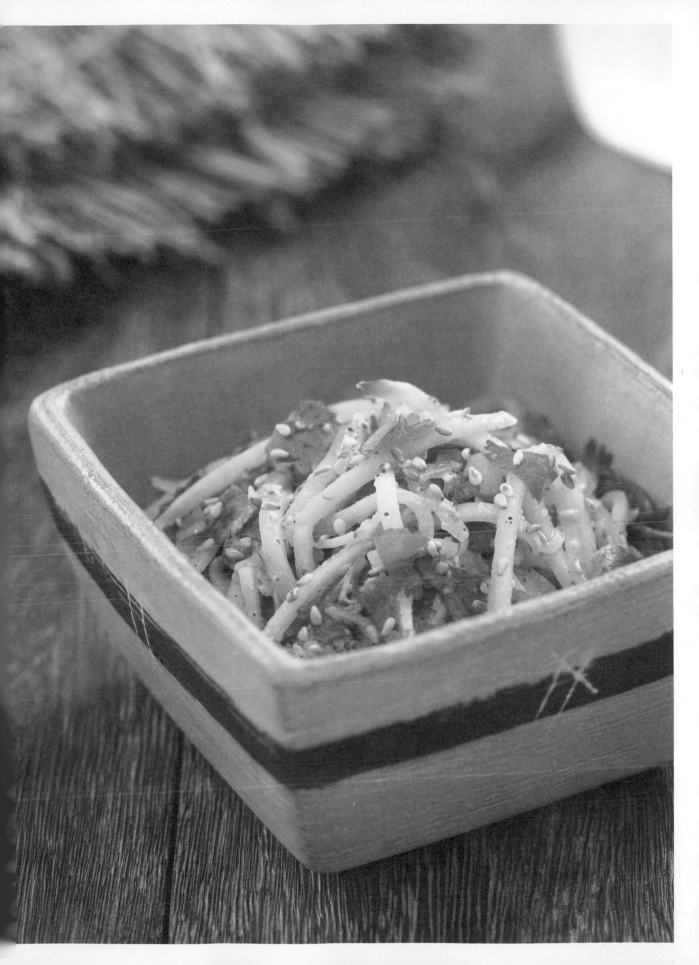

Solomon's Seal

Indigenous to northern Europe and Siberia, Solomon's seal has a creeping root-stock or underground stem that is thick and white, twisted and full of knots, with circular scars at intervals, left by the leaf stems of previous years. The rhizome and herb contain active constituents that are astringent, demulcent and tonic.

Usually sold as slivers of yellowish root at Chinese medicinal shops, the herb is often prescribed in the treatment of ailments of the pancreas and throat. It is said to regulate the lungs and stomach channels, prevent internal dryness, dissipate wind and soften the sinews of the body. Commonly used to treat thirst, muscular cramps and irritability, it is also attributed with aphrodisiac properties. A mucilaginous tonic, the herb is very healing and restorative, and effective in treating inflammations of the bowels, piles and chronic dysentery. The infusion of 30 g (1 oz) of the root in 650 ml (21 fl oz / 2½ cups) boiling water, is often prescribed in wineglassful doses for such ailments.

For external applications, the roots can be ground into a powder and combined in poultices for bruises, piles and tumours. The bruised roots are also used as a popular cure for black (bruised) eyes when mixed with a facial moisturiser and applied on the affected area.

Simmered Pork Soup with Solomon's Seal

Pork is generally regarded as 'cooler' than chicken. It is an ideal ingredient for this slow-simmer dish, which is a real winter warmer. Because of the long cooking process, it is better to cut the pork into large chunks to prevent the meat from drying out.

Preparation time: 20 minutes
Cooking time: 1–1 hour 30 minutes
Serves 4

Lean pork 600 g (1 lb 5 oz), cut into large chunks

Solomon's seal 15 g (½ oz), rinsed and drained

Water 1 litre (32 fl oz / 4 cups)

Salt 2 tsp or more to taste

Combine all ingredients in a pot and simmer for 1–1 hour 30 minutes, depending on the intensity of heat used. Top with hot water as required, if evaporation is rapid and liquid is much reduced.

When ready to serve, taste soup and adjust with more salt, if desired. Serve warm.

Treatments

The astringent properties of Solomon's seal not only make it a fortifying tonic drink, but also useful in a topical poultice for bruises and mild inflammation of the skin. To make an **ointment for minor skin irritations**, grind 30 g (1 oz) of the root using a spice grinder, and blend with just enough almond oil to make a light paste. Apply a thin layer on the affected area, and leave for several hours before rinsing off. For **a treatment for black eyes** and other minor facial wounds such as shaving burns, mix the Solomon's seal paste with some moisturising cream and apply on the affected area. Rinse off after an hour.

Solomon's Seal Tonic Wine

Preparation time: 10 minutes
Cooking time: 20 minutes
Serves 4

Water 400 ml (13 fl oz)

Solomon's seal 60 g (2 oz), blended (processed) into a powder

Ginger wine or Chinese rice wine 400 ml (13 fl oz)

Bring water to the boil, then add Solomon's seal. Remove from heat and allow to steep for 10 minutes, then leave to cool completely.

Blend (process) cooled mixture with ginger or rice wine. Drink it slightly chilled as a rejuvenating tonic.

Note: Ginger wine is a widely available product in most major supermarkets, the most common being Stone's Green Ginger wine, which is also excellent for cooking.

Solomon's Seal, Chrysanthemum and Lotus Seed Tea

This blend is basically 'cooling' and very soothing for sore throats. The infusion of chrysanthemum blooms makes this a very fragrant drink.

Preparation time: 10 minutes
Cooking time: 50 minutes
Serves 4

Solomon's seal 15 g (¹/₂ oz), washed and drained

Rock sugar 150 g (5¹/₃ oz)

Water 1.5 litres (48 fl oz / 6 cups)

Precooked lotus seeds 40

Dried chrysanthemum flowers 50 g (2 oz)

Combine Solomon's seal, rock sugar and water in a pot. Bring to the boil and simmer for 40 minutes.

Add lotus seeds and chrysanthemum flowers. Simmer for 10 minutes more before serving warm.

FROM LEFT TO RIGHT: Solomon's Seal, Chrysanthemum and Lotus Seed Tea (page 158), Treatment: Ointment for Minor Skin Irritations (page 157), Solomon's Seal Tonic Wine (page 158)

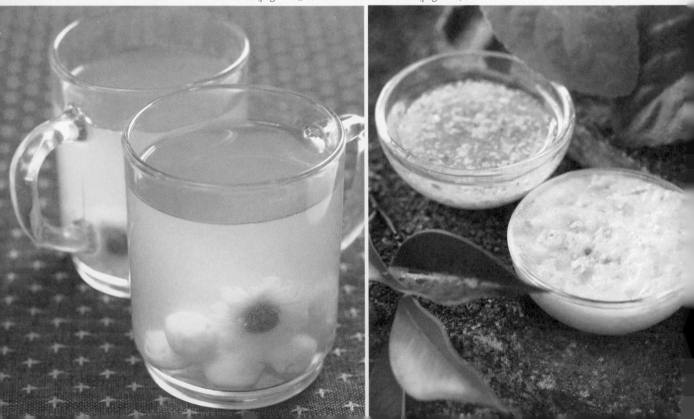

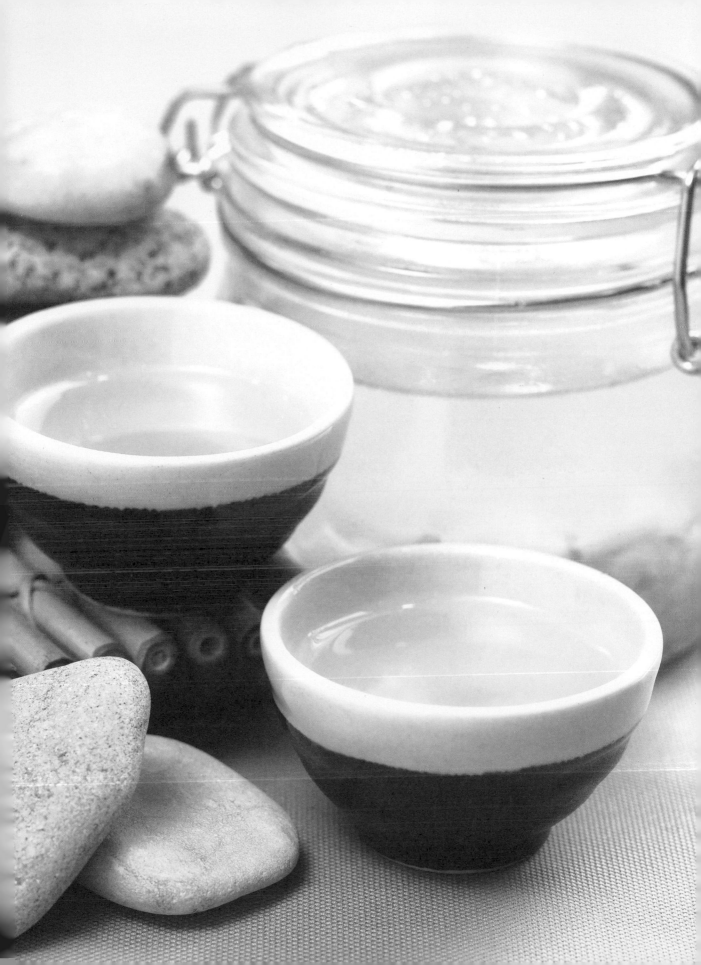

Sterculia Seed

Common Sterculia seed
Mandarin Pang da hai
Cantonese Dai hau lahm
Botanical Sterculia scaphigera semen

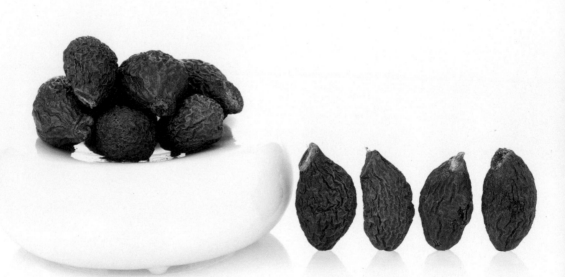

The seed, despite its name, is actually a kind of fruit. Sold dried at Chinese herbal shops, it expands at an alarming rate when soaked in water. Its Mandarin name literally means 'fat big ocean'. It is rather like white fungus in taste, and often used in the hawker's sweet drink, *ngo bee tng* or five-flavoured soup.

Medicinally, the sterculia seed has properties for clearing the lungs and bowels, as well as moistening the throat. It is also effective in treating heaty phlegm, constipation and fever.

Black Chicken Soup with Chinese Angelica and Sterculia Seed

Although generally associated with desserts, I often use sterculia seed in a savoury dish such as this. Black on black is intriguing and this blend with angelica does one a power of good. Black chicken has, for centuries in China, been deemed superior to ordinary birds for their restorative properties.

Preparation time: 20 minutes
Cooking time: 1 hour
Serves 4

Sterculia seed 1

Black chicken 650 g (1 lb 7 oz), cleaned and cut into 4 joints, or leave whole as desired

Chinese angelica 30 g (1 oz), rinsed and drained

Water 1 litre (32 fl oz / 4 cups)

Salt 2 tsp

Soak sterculia seed in ample water for 10 minutes, or until slightly softened. Make a slit in the skin along one side of the seed so that water can penetrate and hydrate the flesh. Soak for 10 minutes more, or until flesh has expanded into a loose, jellylike mass. Peel off and discard the thin skin.

Put all ingredients into a pot and bring to the boil, then reduce heat and simmer for 45 minutes or until chicken is tender.

Remove and discard all herbs. Serve warm.

Lotus Seeds, Sweet Potatoes and Sterculia Seed

Sterculia seeds for me, will always bring back memories of my *ngo bee tng* or five-flavoured soup hawker in Singapore, who used them liberally in a range of hot desserts.

Preparation time: 15 minutes
Cooking time: 45 minutes
Serves 4

Sterculia seed 1

Water 1 litre (32 fl oz / 4 cups)

Rock sugar 150 g (5 1/3 oz) or more to taste

Sweet potatoes 300 g (10 2/3 oz), peeled, cut into 1.5-cm (0.75-in) dice, washed and drained

Precooked lotus seeds 250 g (9 oz)

Soak sterculia seed in ample water for 10 minutes, or until slightly softened. Make a slit in the skin along one side of the seed so that water can penetrate and hydrate the flesh. Soak for 10 minutes more, or until flesh has expanded into a loose, jellylike mass. Peel off and discard the thin skin.

Bring water to the boil in a pot. Add rock sugar and sweet potatoes and simmer for 15 minutes, until sweet potatoes are cooked.

Add lotus and sterculia seeds and simmer 2 minutes more. Taste and adjust sugar, if desired. Serve warm as a dessert.

Lotus Seeds, Sweet Potatoes and Sterculia Seed (page 161)

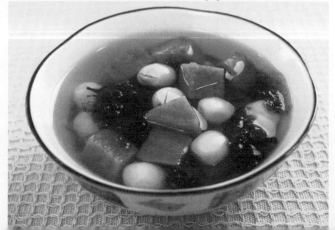

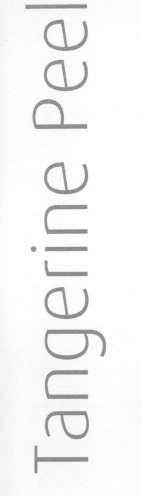

Tangerine Peel

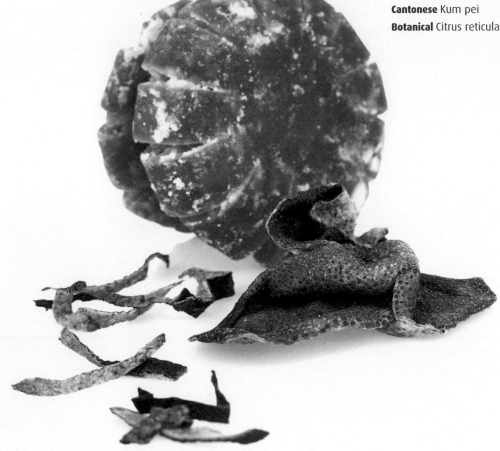

Common Tangerine peel
Mandarin Chen pi
Cantonese Kum pei
Botanical Citrus reticulate

The Chinese have been using dried citrus peel as a therapeutic herb for centuries, with tangerine peels being the most widely consumed because of the relative ease in obtaining them.

Sour, bitter and pungent in character, the constituents of the fruit peel are volatile oil, vitamins A, B and C, flavanoids and bitters. Tangerine peel has carminative, digestive, antiseptic, anti-spasmodic and anti-depressant qualities that help regulate blood pressure; it also serves as an expectorant for dispelling phlegm in coughs and is highly effective as an energy tonic. Traditionally, soups and drinks infused with the essence of tangerine peel are prescribed for coughs, colds and dyspepsia, and also act as antidotes for poisoning from the consumption of fish. Known as *qing pi*, meaning literally 'green skin' in Mandarin, the dried peel of young or unripe tangerines are also used in TCM, in combination with other herbs for many common ailments including low blood pressure.

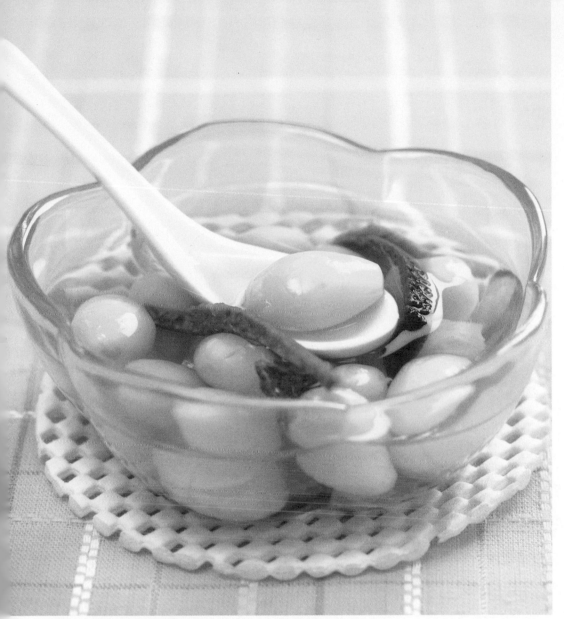
Gingko Nuts with Tangerine Peel (page 163)

Gingko Nuts with Tangerine Peel

Gingko nuts are known for their antioxidant and anti-allergic properties to improve circulation and enhance energy metabolism in the brain. Combined with tangerine peel, this makes a warming drink that helps to dispel phlegm and also aid digestion.

Preparation time: 10 minutes
Cooking time: 30 minutes
Serves 4

Water 1.5 litres (48 fl oz / 6 cups)

Precooked gingko nuts 40

Dried tangerine peel 4–5 strips, each about 3-cm (1.5-in) long

Rock sugar 150 g (5 1/3 oz)

Bring water to the boil in a pot. Add remaining ingredients and simmer over medium-low heat for 30 minutes. Add more water, if required.

Serve warm or chilled, as a dessert.

Note: If you are using dried gingko nuts, soak them overnight and remove bitter cores by pushing them through the nuts with a toothpick before using. Cooking time will vary, depending on how soft the nuts are.

Pork Soup with Peanuts and Tangerine Peel

This is a hearty and delicious soup, of which you can consume bowls of, as it has the subtlest flavour, using tangerine peel as the only herb in the dish.

Preparation time: 20 minutes
Cooking time: 1 hour
Serves 4

Lean pork 600 g (1 lb 5 oz), cut into bite-sized chunks

Shelled raw peanuts 200 g (7 oz)

Dried tangerine peel 30 g (1 oz)

Water 1.5 litres (48 fl oz / 6 cups)

Salt 2 tsp

Ground black pepper 1 tsp

Combine all ingredients in a pot and simmer for 1 hour or longer, if you prefer fork-tender pork.

Remove and discard tangerine peel before serving hot with rice and other dishes, if desired.

Note: Substitute with chicken, which tastes just as good, if desired.

Skinned Duck with Dried Apricots and Tangerine Peel

Dried fruits have been a Chinese mainstay for centuries, and not simply as a winter snack, but used liberally in cooking. Duck, with its oily richness, is particularly suited to fruits, whether dried or fresh.

Preparation time: 30 minutes
Cooking time: 1 hour 30 minutes
Serves 6

Duck 1, about 2 kg (4 lb 6 oz), thoroughly cleaned, skinned and cut into large joints

Dried apricots 6

Garlic 4 cloves, peeled and left whole

Dried tangerine peel 4 pieces, 3-cm (1.5-in) wide strips

Salt 2 tsp

Water 2 litres (64 fl oz / 8 cups)

Combine all ingredients in a pot and simmer for 1 hour 30 minutes. At the end of cooking time, the liquid in pot should have reduced by about half.

Serve hot with rice and other dishes, if desired.

Note: This recipe can be pressure-cooked, which means that the amount of water can be reduced by as much as half, as long as there is sufficient liquid in the pot to cover all the duck joints.

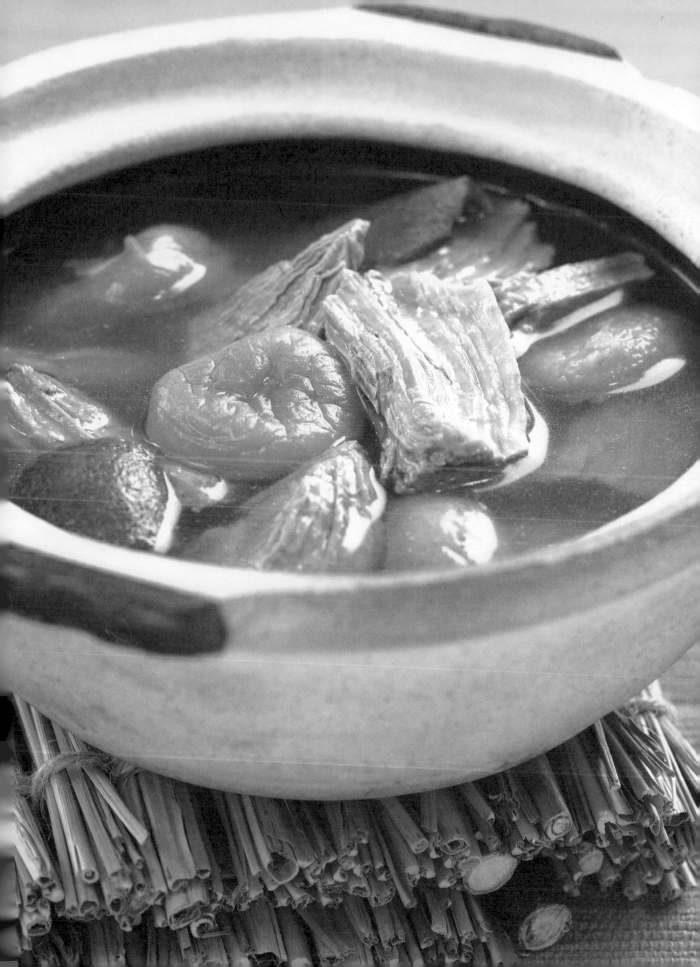

Tea

Common Tea
Mandarin Cha
Cantonese Cha
Botanical Camellia sinensis

What has not been written about this quintessentially Chinese leaf in the 3,000 years that it has dominated the world? It is drunk by virtually the whole of humanity — a universal panacea and getting better known each day as a medicinal herb rather than just as a beverage.

Basically of three types — green, black and oolong — each tea has specific characteristics. Green and oolong teas are bittersweet and cooling, while black tea is bitter and cooling. All are leaves from the same plant species which have constituents of caffeine, tannins and volatile oil, with stimulant, astringent, antioxidant, antibacterial and diuretic actions.

Research has also shown that green tea helps to reduce blood cholesterol levels, combat stomach and skin cancers as well as boost the immune system. With its potent antibacterial qualities, green tea has unique powers in dealing with common skin ailments like acne and eczema. Green tea has also been reported to help in healing wounds and minimising the scarring of tissue; the polyphenol in green tea possesses the ability to reactivate cells in the outer dermis. Oolong tea varieties such as *pu erh,* are regarded as effective in cutting down fat and reducing high blood pressure. Often prescribed for diarrhoea, black tea is rich in tannins and is highly astringent.

Ginger and Lemon Grass Tea

This is a very soothing tea and goes very well with spicy Thai food.

Preparation time: 15 minutes
Cooking time: 10 minutes
Serves 4

Water 800 ml (26 fl oz / 3¼ cups)

Lemon grass 3 stalks, use lower ends only, lightly bruised

Ginger 1 knob, 80 g (3 oz), peeled and bruised

Earl Grey tea bags 2

Lemon slices

Honey to taste

Bring water to the boil in a pot. Add lemon grass and ginger. Simmer for 15 minutes.

Strain liquid and discard solids. Return liquid to the boil, then remove from heat, add tea bags and leave to steep for 5 minutes.

Strain tea and serve warm with lemon slices and honey to taste.

Tea Eggs

When I first learnt how to do tea eggs from a grand master chef who was visiting the cookery institute run by the late Ken Lo, and where I was teaching, I fell in love with these beautifully marbled eggs. For me, marbled quail eggs are such an amusing starter — they are ever so simple to make, and a wonderful talking point at parties.

Preparation time: 10 minutes
Cooking time: 45 minutes
Serves 4

Chicken eggs 8

Cooking Liquid

Black tea leaves 2 Tbsp

Water for tea 1 litre (32 fl oz / 4 cups)

Star anise 3

Dark soy sauce 2 Tbsp

Salt 2 tsp

Place eggs in a pot of cold water to fully cover and bring to the boil. Cook for 10 minutes.

Tap each egg gently all over with the back of a metal spoon to make a fine, irregular network of cracks all over.

Put all ingredients for cooking liquid and boiled eggs into a deep pot and bring to the boil. Reduce heat to low, partially cover and simmer for 1 hour. Remove eggs with a slotted spoon and let cool on a plate completely.

When cool, shell eggs and serve. Each egg will be delicately marbled.

Note: You can use quail, chicken or duck eggs for this recipe.

Green Tea Ice Cream

Preparation time: 35 minutes
Cooking time: 10 minutes
Serves 4

Hot water 70 ml (2^1/$_3$ fl oz)

Green tea powder 3 Tbsp

Whipping cream, chilled 400 ml (13^1/$_3$ fl oz / 1^7/$_8$ cups)

Egg whites 2

Icing sugar 100 g (3^1/$_2$ oz)

In a medium bowl, slowly whisk hot water into green tea powder to make a thick paste. Let cool completely.

In a large mixing bowl, whisk whipping cream until thick, floppy and just about to stiffen. Cover and set aside in the coldest part of the fridge.

Combine egg whites and icing sugar in a separate metal mixing bowl. Set bowl over a pot of barely simmering water — to keep temperature constant, be careful not to let bottom of bowl touch the water. Stir with a whisk until sugar has dissolved and egg whites are very warm to the touch, then beat until a stiff-peaked meringue forms, 2–3 minutes. Remove from heat.

Remove whipped cream from fridge and scrape cooled tea paste into mixture, then gently fold in with a whisk. Add half the meringue and fold in until almost even. Add remaining meringue and fold only until just incorporated.

Spoon mixture into an airtight container, cover and freeze for at least 5 hours until firm. For a smoother texture, alternately freeze and beat ice cream briefly at half-hourly intervals after the first hour of freezing for up to 4 hours. Serve as desired.

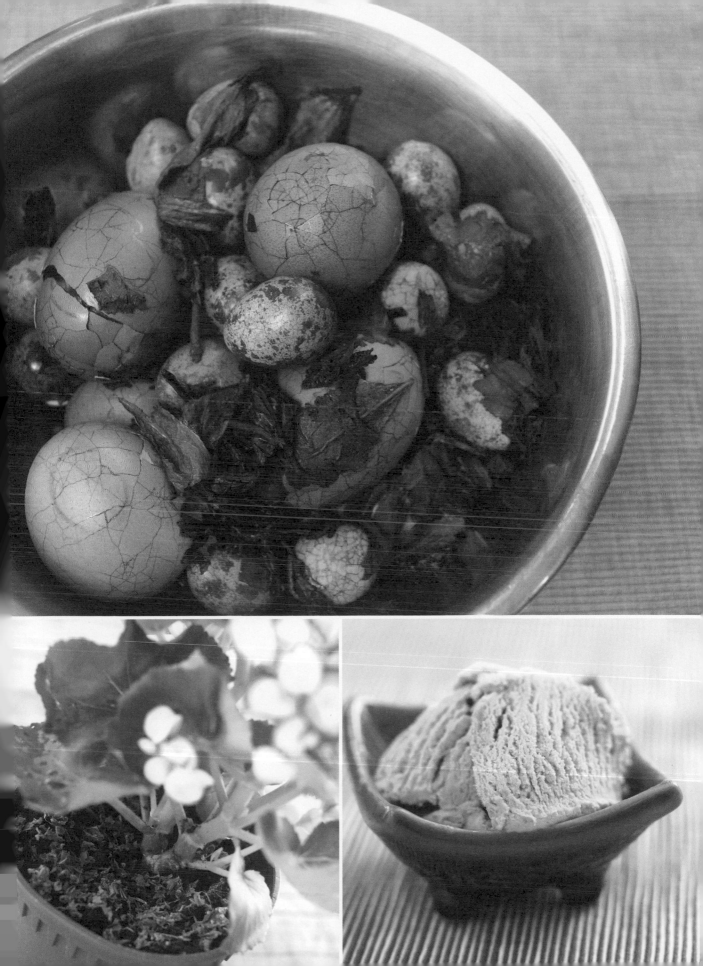

Tea-Smoked Chicken

Why stop at brewing tea purely as a drink? The smoky essence of *pu er* or *tie kuan yin* lends itself aromatically to chicken and duck. It is fairly easy to rig your own 'smoker' as it were, although this dish is actually oven-cooked.

Preparation time: 20 minutes
Cooking time: 1 hour
Serves 4

Chicken 1, about 1.5 kg (3 lb 4¹/₂ oz), cleaned, trimmed of excess fat and pat dry

Salt 2 tsp

Coarsly ground black pepper 2 tsp

Sugar 1 Tbsp

***Pu er* tea leaves** 2 Tbsp

Sesame oil 2 Tbsp

Rub chicken all over with salt and pepper.

Prepare a double-layer sheet of aluminium foil, large enough to line roasting pan, with excess on both sides to fold over and cover chicken completely.

Line roasting pan with foil sheet, then sprinkle sugar and tea leaves all over. Set a roasting rack over mixture of tea leaves and place chicken on rack.

Fold both sides of aluminium foil to cover chicken completely and secure. Put roasting pan into a preheated oven at 200°C (400°F) and roast for 35 minutes.

Unwrap chicken and brush with sesame oil, then return to oven and roast, uncovered, for a further 20 minutes until golden brown.

Allow chicken to rest for 15 minutes before carving into serving pieces. Serve warm with rice and other dishes, if desired.

Treatments

Do not throw away used tea bags as they are very useful in rejuvenating tired eyes. For a **soothing eye treatment**, simply chill tea bags for about half an hour, then place one over each eye for 15 minutes before discarding.

To make a green tea compress, soak a thick wad of cotton wool in green tea, then squeeze lightly and apply to minor cuts and bruises for 10–15 minutes before removing. Repeat once or twice a day.

To make a poultice for treating insect bites and minor skin irritations, boil 3 Tbsp green tea leaves in 500 ml (16 fl oz / 2 cups) water for 4 minutes. Squeeze out excess moisture from tea leaves and when cool to the touch, apply tea leaves to the skin. Wrap with clean cotton gauze to keep the poultice in place for several hours, until itch and swell subside.

To neutralise any bad odour in the fridge, fill a thin cotton bag with green tea leaves and leave it in the fridge. The filled bag can also be added to the final wash for chopping boards to remove any fishy or strong odours.

Treat your potted plants with **natural green tea fertiliser** — simply scatter a thin layer of used green tea leaves on the surface soil around the plants, and they will be sure to reward you with shiny new leaves.

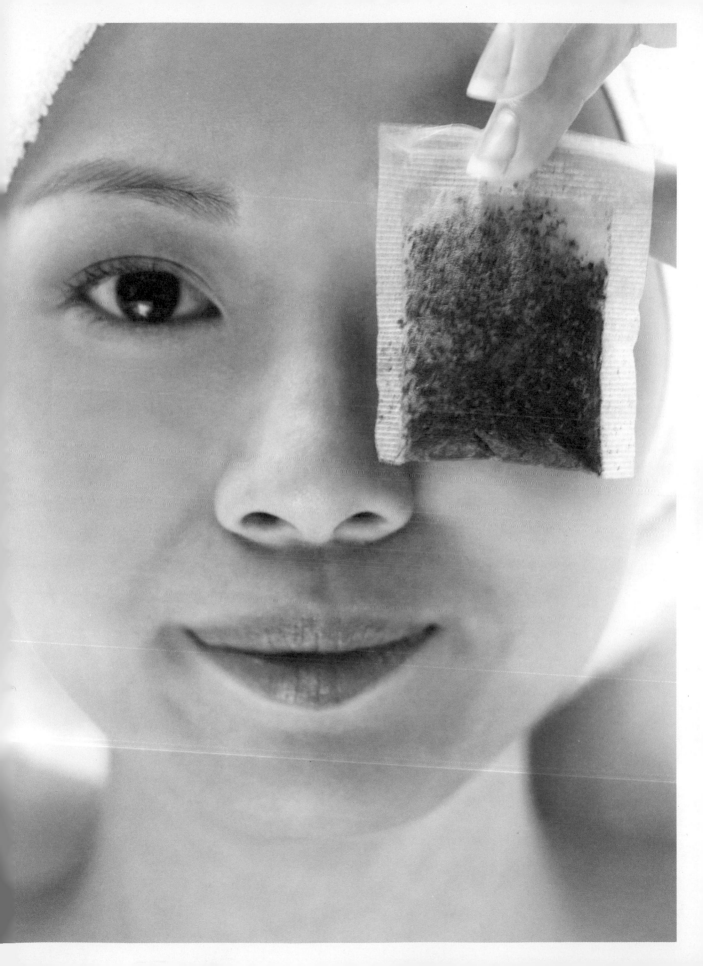

Common Turmeric
Mandarin Yu jin
Cantonese Wong keong
Botanical Curcuma longa

In both Chinese herbalism and Indian Ayurvedic applications, turmeric has long been considered effective for the treatment of ailments such as arthritis, inflammation of the muscles, skin rashes and physical pain. Hot and dry in nature, it is used both internally and externally as a medicine, like many other spices.

With powerful antioxidants that influence heart, liver and lung functions, turmeric also improves blood circulation and the flow of Qi in the body, and regulates the gall bladder and bladder functions at the same time.

It is the root of the plant that contains the primary ingredient, curcumin, which helps one to maintain a healthy digestive system and regulate bowel function. Turmeric is also available in tablet form, but should not be taken in high doses as it increases the flow of bile in the body.

Stir-fried Prawns with Tropical Herbs (page 174)

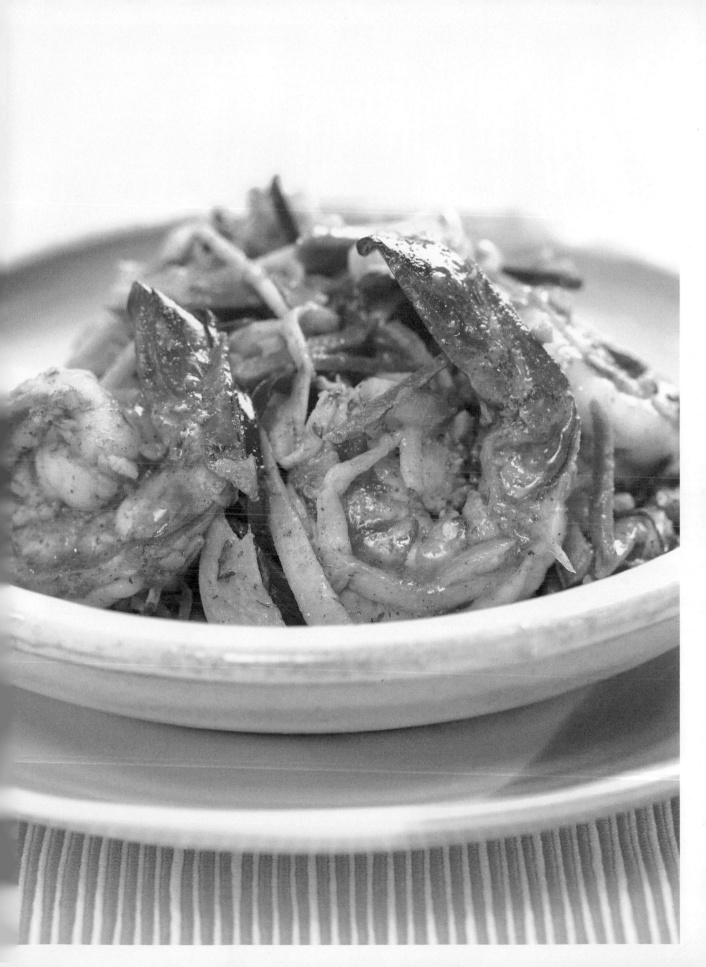

Stir-fried Prawns with Tropical Herbs

This is a rich mélange of flavours in a moist unusual blend of aromatic flavours from fresh herbs like turmeric, galangal, lemon grass, chillies and garlic.

Preparation time: 20 minutes
Cooking time: 10 minutes
Serves 4

Cooking oil 2 Tbsp

Ginger 20 g ($^2/_3$ oz), peeled and sliced

Turmeric 20 g ($^2/_3$ oz), peeled and sliced

Galangal 15 g ($^1/_2$ oz), peeled and sliced

Red chillies 4, seeded and finely julienned

Shallots 6, peeled and thinly sliced

Garlic 4 cloves, peeled and thinly sliced

Tiger prawns (shrimps) 16, deveined and shelled, but with tails left intact, and cleaned

Preserved soy beans (*tau cheo*) 1 Tbsp, lightly mashed

Sugar 2 tsp

Lime juice 2 Tbsp

Water 3 Tbsp

Heat oil in a wok. Add ginger, turmeric, galangal, chillies, shallots and garlic and fry for 2 minutes until light brown.

Increase heat and add prawns, preserved soy beans, sugar and lime juice. Stir-fry over high heat until prawns are cooked.

Add water and bring to a quick boil. Remove from heat and dish out. Serve hot with rice and other dishes.

Turmeric Fish

This is a modified version of a richer northern Malaysian dish called *percik* that usually uses chicken, but the spice blend is the same.

Threadfin (*ikan kurau*), 500 g (1 lb 1$^1/_2$ oz), cut into thick steaks

Coconut cream 3 Tbsp

Lemon juice 1 Tbsp

Cumin powder 1 Tbsp

Coriander powder 1 Tbsp

Turmeric powder 1 tsp

Finely ground black pepper 1 tsp

Salt 1 tsp

Cooking oil 2 Tbsp

Wash and pat fish dry. Blend all other ingredients except cooking oil and rub all over fish. Cover and marinate in the fridge for at least 1 hour.

Brush fish steaks with oil. Place under a pre-heated grill and cook for 6–8 minutes on each side, until brown and crisp, turning once.

Serve hot with rice and other dishes.

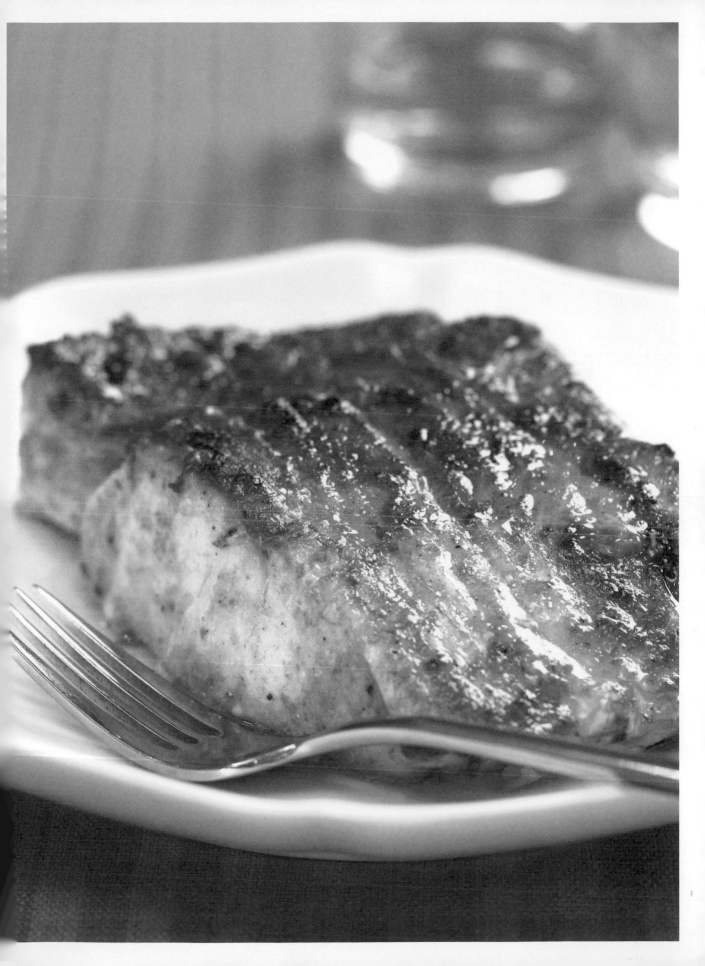

White Fungus

Common White fungus
Mandarin Bai mu er
Cantonese Shuet yi
Botanical Tremella fuciformis

Often confused with the more expensive and entirely different product called hasma or *shuet kup* in Cantonese, which refers to the dried glands of the northern snow frog, white fungus is similar in form to black fungus, which is commonly known as wood ears or *mok yi* in Cantonese.

Herbalists sell white fungus dried, and the hard pieces are yellowish-brown in colour. The fungus regains its white colour when soaked in water to soften before use. A neutral product, white fungus influences the functions of the stomach and lungs and is known to nourish nutritive fluids in the body and whet appetite. It is also taken to alleviate dry coughs and bloody phlegm.

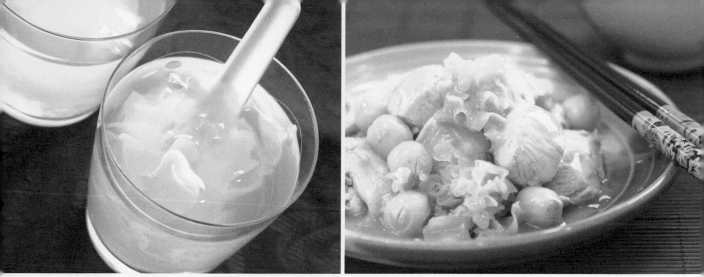

FROM LEFT TO RIGHT: *White Fungus Drink (page 177), Stir-fried Chicken with White Fungus and Lotus Seeds (page 177)*

Stir-fried Chicken with White Fungus and Lotus Seeds

Although it has relatively little taste, white fungus has a crunchy texture in a stir-fry which I like.

Preparation time: 15 minutes
Cooking time: 15 minutes
Serves 4

White fungus 30 g (1 oz), soaked in warm water to rehydrate, and drained

Cooking oil 2 Tbsp

Chopped garlic 1 Tbsp

Chicken breast 400 g (14 oz), cut into 2-cm (1-in) dice

Water 150 ml (5 fl oz / 5/8 cup)

Precooked lotus seeds 20

Salt 2 tsp

Chopped garlic 1 Tbsp

Sesame oil 2 Tbsp

Light soy sauce 1 Tbsp

Corn flour (cornstarch) 1 Tbsp, mixed with 2 Tbsp water

Trim and discard hard bits of white fungus, cut into small pieces, then wash and drain.

Heat oil and fry garlic for 2 minutes until golden brown.

Add chicken and stir-fry over high heat for 2 minutes, then add white fungus, water and lotus seeds. Simmer for 3 minutes until chicken is thoroughly cooked.

Add remaining ingredients except cornflour mixture and simmer for 1 minute. Finally, stir in cornflour mixture to thicken sauce slightly.

Remove from heat, then dish out and serve hot with rice and other dishes.

White Fungus Drink

Also known as white tremella mushroom, this gelatinous ingredient is delicious and delightfully crunchy in a sweet or savoury soup.

Preparation time: 10 minutes
Cooking time: 45 minutes
Serves 4

White fungus 60 g (2 oz), soaked in warm water to rehydrate, and drained

Water 1 litre (32 fl oz / 1 cup)

Rock sugar 150 g (5 1/3 oz)

Screwpine (*pandan*) leaves 2, washed and knotted

Trim and discard hard bits of white fungus, cut into small pieces, then wash and drain.

Combine all ingredients in a pot. Simmer for 45 minutes or until fungus is almost jellied. Remove and discard screwpine leaves.

Serve warm or chilled. It will glide down your throat like no other herbal drink does.

Winter Melon

Common Winter melon
Mandarin Dong gua
Cantonese Tung kwa
Botanical Benicasa hispida

Winter melon rind, dried and sugared, is a popular traditional sweet in some cultures. A native of tropical Asia and widely grown in many countries, the fresh fruit is probably the most widely-known variety of melon.

In China, all parts of the fruit, including the seeds, rind, pulp and juice of the melon, are regarded as medicinal. While the whole fruit has diuretic qualities, its seeds are used as a mild laxative as well as a tonic, and are believed to be good for the treatment of haemorrhoids, intestinal inflammation, urinary and kidney diseases, diabetes and dropsy. The flesh of the fruit, when boiled with rock sugar, is believed to be exceptionally 'cooling' for the body. For external application, the ash of the rind is applied directly onto painful wounds because of its antiseptic and analgesic properties.

Stir-Fried Winter Melon, Chicken and Gingko Nuts

Yes, you can stir-fry winter melon and, in fact, it is rather like a root vegetable, but softer in texture. The contrast in texture comes from the gingko nuts; altogether, a perfect Yin Yang blend.

Preparation time: 10 minutes
Cooking time: 10 minutes
Serves 4

Cooking oil 2 Tbsp

Garlic 2 cloves, peeled and crushed

Chicken breast 200 g (7 oz), cut into thick matchsticks

Winter melon 250 g (9 oz), peeled, pith removed and cut into matchsticks

Precooked gingko nuts 20–30

Salt 2 tsp

Sesame oil 2 Tbsp

Water 100 ml (3 1/3 fl oz / 3/8 cup)

Chopped coriander leaves 2 Tbsp

Heat oil in a wok and fry garlic for 1 minute until light brown. Add chicken and stir-fry over high heat for 2 minutes.

Add winter melon, gingko nuts and salt, then stir-fry for 1 minute. Add sesame oil and water and bring to a brisk boil for 3 minutes. Remove from heat.

Dish out and garnish with fresh coriander. Serve hot with rice and other dishes.

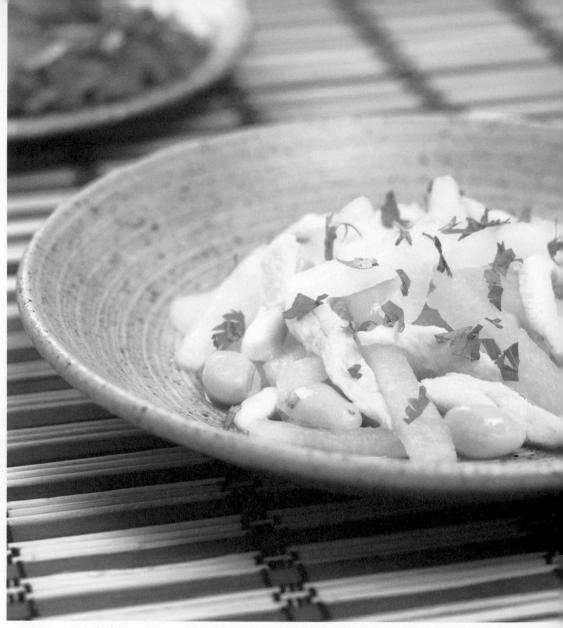

FROM LEFT TO RIGHT: Stir-fried Winter Melon, Chicken and Gingko Nuts (page 179), Winter Melon, Pork and Lotus Seed Soup (page 180)

Winter Melon, Pork and Lotus Seed Soup

Winter melon is known for its cooling properties and this combination jacks up its Yin potential even more. Pork is a largely neutral meat and considered 'cool' as well.

Preparation time: 10 minutes
Cooking time: 30 minutes
Serves 4

Water 1 litre (32 fl oz / 4 cups)

Lean pork 200 g (7 oz), thinly sliced or julienned

Winter melon flesh 200 g (7 oz), cut into 1-cm ($^1/_2$-in) dice

Precooked lotus seeds 20–30

Light soy sauce 1 Tbsp

Ground white pepper 1 tsp

Bring water to the boil in a pot. Add pork and winter melon. Bring to the boil, then reduce heat and simmer over medium-low heat for 30 minutes.

Add lotus seeds, soy sauce and pepper. Cook for 5 minutes more. Serve hot.

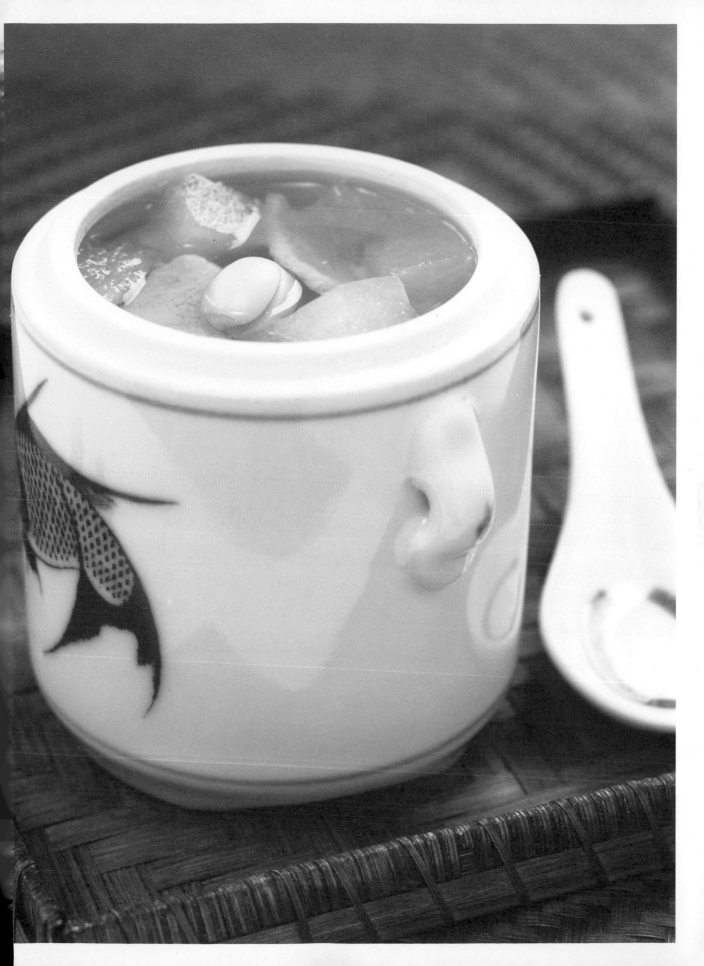

Wood Ear Fungus

Common Wood ear fungus
Mandarin Mu erh
Cantonese Mook yee
Botanical Auricularia Polytricha

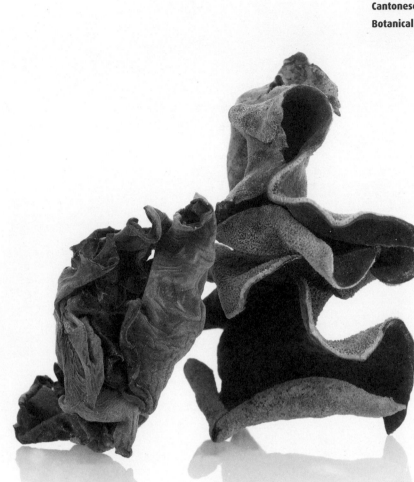

Variously known as tree ears, dried black fungus and silver ears, wood ear mushrooms are cultivated all over the world but grown for commercial purposes almost exclusively in western China. Typically sold dried, they are also available fresh nowadays, and are popular both as a food and as herbal medicine.

The fungus looks like ears growing out of trees, hence its name — with flat, plate-like caps that can reach 20 cm (8-in) across. It is often confused with the cloud ear mushroom; they are similar in appearance except that wood ear fungus is black with a brownish-tan inner colour, and it assumes a striking silver-black contrast when dried.

Fresh wood ear fungus has a firm, thick skin and a spongy, springy yet soft texture that becomes slightly crunchy when cooked. Medicinally, the fungus is believed by many to prevent heart disease and to lower blood pressure. It contains substances that are anti-coagulant, and act as blood thinners for preventing the blood from clotting — similar to an aspirin.

Stir-fried Wood Ear Fungus with Assorted Vegetables

This famous dish, in its full glory with 18 varieties of vegetables, is known as 'the 18 Lohan', to symbolise the 18 disciples of the Lord Buddha. However, it is just as tasty and healthy with fewer vegetables as in this adapted recipe. Based on the philosophy of Chinese cooking, each vegetable has its own efficacy for better health, or reflects positive symbolism. Celery, for instance, promotes better circulation while mushrooms, apart from symbolising wealth, are also low in fat and high in essential nutrients.

Preparation time: 20 minutes
Cooking time: 25 minutes
Serves 8

Cooking oil 2 Tbsp

Crushed garlic 2 Tbsp

Preserved red bean curd (nam yee) 2 Tbsp

Celery 2 stalks, sliced diagonally into 2-cm (1-in) lengths

Wood ear fungus 50 g (2 oz), soaked in water to rehydrate, hard bits trimmed off and cut into small pieces, then washed and drained

Canned or precooked bamboo shoot 75 g (2½ oz), sliced into 2-cm (1-in) wide pieces

Red capsicum 1, seeded and sliced into 2-cm (1-in) wide pieces

Chinese napa cabbage (bak choy) 75 g (2½ oz), sliced into 2-cm (1-in) wide pieces

Hoi sin sauce 1 Tbsp

Light soy sauce 1 Tbsp

Oyster sauce 2 Tbsp

Water 400 ml (13⅓ fl oz)

Heat oil and stir-fry garlic until light brown. Add preserved red bean curd and crush with spatula.

Add all vegetables and stir-fry over high heat for 2 minutes. Mix well. Add remaining ingredients and simmer over medium–low heat for 20 minutes, until vegetables are cooked. Remove from heat.

Dish out and serve hot with rice and other dishes.

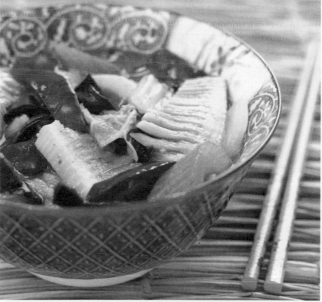

Stir-fried Wood Ear Fungus with Assorted Vegetables (page 183)

Weights and Measures

Quantities for this book are given in Metric, Imperial and American (spoon) measures.
Standard spoon and cup measurements used are:
1 tsp = 5 ml, 1 Tbsp = 15 ml, 1 cup = 250 ml. All measures are level unless otherwise stated.

LIQUID AND VOLUME MEASURES

Metric	Imperial	American
5 ml	$1/6$ fl oz	1 teaspoon
10 ml	$1/3$ fl oz	1 dessertspoon
15 ml	$1/2$ fl oz	1 tablespoon
60 ml	2 fl oz	$1/4$ cup (4 tablespoons)
85 ml	$2^1/2$ fl oz	$1/3$ cup
90 ml	3 fl oz	$3/8$ cup (6 tablespoons)
125 ml	4 fl oz	$1/2$ cup
180 ml	6 fl oz	$3/4$ cup
250 ml	8 fl oz	1 cup
300 ml	10 fl oz ($1/2$ pint)	$1^1/4$ cups
375 ml	12 fl oz	$1^1/2$ cups
435 ml	14 fl oz	$1^3/4$ cups
500 ml	16 fl oz	2 cups
625 ml	20 fl oz (1 pint)	$2^1/2$ cups
750 ml	24 fl oz ($1^1/5$ pints)	3 cups
1 litre	32 fl oz ($1^3/5$ pints)	4 cups
1.25 litres	40 fl oz (2 pints)	5 cups
1.5 litres	48 fl oz ($2^2/5$ pints)	6 cups
2.5 litres	80 fl oz (4 pints)	10 cups

DRY MEASURES

Metric	Imperial
30 grams	1 ounce
45 grams	$1^1/2$ ounces
55 grams	2 ounces
70 grams	$2^1/2$ ounces
85 grams	3 ounces
100 grams	$3^1/2$ ounces
110 grams	4 ounces
125 grams	$4^1/2$ ounces
140 grams	5 ounces
280 grams	10 ounces
450 grams	16 ounces (1 pound)
500 grams	1 pound, $1^1/2$ ounces
700 grams	$1^1/2$ pounds
800 grams	$1^3/4$ pounds
1 kilogram	2 pounds, 3 ounces
1.5 kilograms	3 pounds, $4^1/2$ ounces
2 kilograms	4 pounds, 6 ounces

LENGTH

Metric	Imperial
0.5 cm	$1/4$ inch
1 cm	$1/2$ inch
1.5 cm	$3/4$ inch
2.5 cm	1 inch

OVEN TEMPERATURE

	°C	°F	Gas Regulo
Very slow	120	250	1
Slow	150	300	2
Moderately slow	160	325	3
Moderate	180	350	4
Moderately hot	190/200	370/400	5/6
Hot	210/220	410/440	6/7
Very hot	230	450	8
Super hot	250/290	475/550	9/10

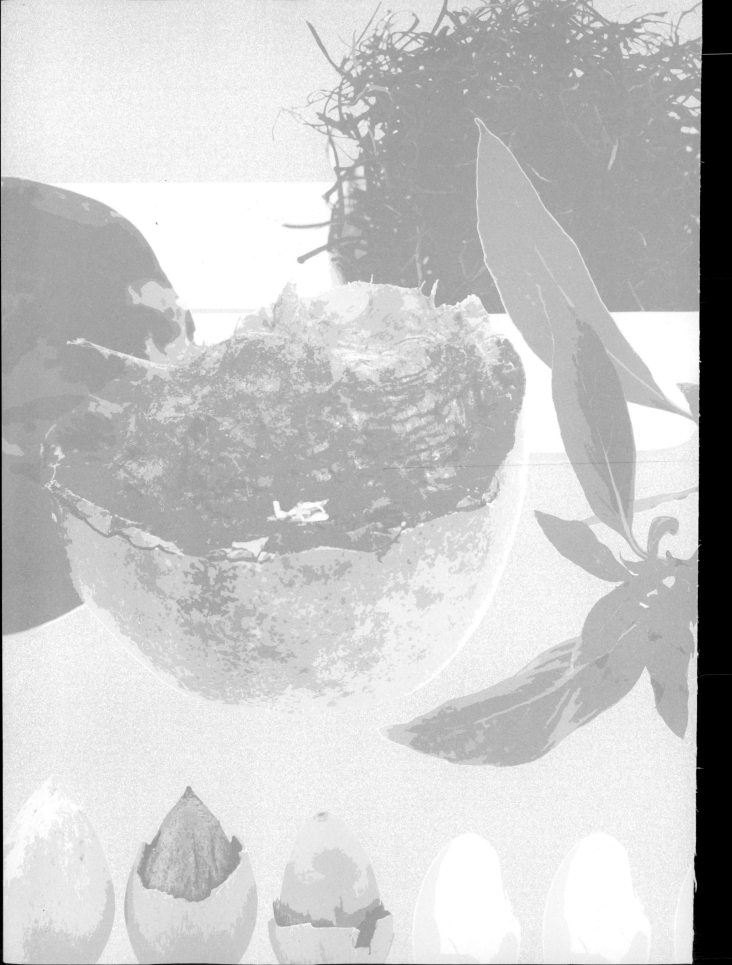